Dream Sociometry

This unique book is the first of two volumes that describe a new, transpersonal model for therapeutic work on dreams. *Dream Sociometry*, a form of Integral Deep Listening (IDL) life drama and dream character interviewing, contributes to the fields of application of the sociometric methods of J. L. Moreno and the use of sociometry in therapy to support and direct personal development. The book describes an experiential, multi-perspectival integral life practice through accessing "emerging potentials," or perspectives that integrate, transcend, and include one's current context and predicament.

Dream Sociometry provides a thoroughly phenomenological approach, suspending interpretation as well as assumptions about the reality and usefulness of synchronicities, mystical experiences, waking accidents, dreams, and nightmares in favor of listening to dream characters and personifications of important life issues in a respectful and integral way. It thereby provides an important doorway to both causal and non-dual awareness by accessing perspectives that personify both, and will open doors for those interested not only in dream research, but in reducing anxiety disorders, such as phobias and post-traumatic stress disorders, and seeing through the often literal and concrete interpretations that we often give both physical and mental illness as well as mystical experiences.

Offering a fresh and unique approach to both dreamwork and self-development through sociometric methodologies, this book will be of interest to researchers in the fields of psychodrama, sociometry, group psychotherapy, transpersonal, experiential, and action therapies, as well as postgraduate students studying psychology and sociology.

Joseph Dillard is a psychotherapist and author of over 20 books on transpersonal development. He is the creator of Integral Deep Listening, a multi-perspectival integral life practice.

Also by Joseph Dillard

Dream Sociometry

A Multi-Perspectival Path to the Transpersonal

Joseph Dillard

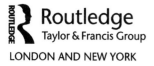

Routledge
Taylor & Francis Group

LONDON AND NEW YORK

First published 2018 by Routledge

2 Park Square, Milton Park, Abingdon, Oxfordshire OX14 4RN
52 Vanderbilt Avenue, New York, NY 10017

Routledge is an imprint of the Taylor & Francis Group, an informa business

First issued in paperback 2020

British Library Cataloguing-in-Publication Data
A catalogue record for this book is available from the British
Library

Library of Congress Cataloging-in-Publication Data
Names: Dillard, Joseph, author.
Title: Dream sociometry: a multi-perspectival path to the
    transpersonal Joseph Dillard.
Description: Milton Park, Abingdon, Oxon ; New York, NY :
    Routledge, 2018. | Includes bibliographical references and index.
Identifiers: LCCN 2017054784 (print) | LCCN 2017056034 (ebook) |
    ISBN 9781351137461 (E-book) | ISBN 9780815353065 (hbk) |
    ISBN 9781351137461 (ebk)
Subjects: LCSH: Dreams—Therapeutic use. | Transpersonal
    psychology.
Classification: LCC RC489.D74 (ebook) | LCC RC489.D74 D55
    2018 (print) | DDC 612.8/21—dc23
LC record available at https://lccn.loc.gov/2017054784

ISBN: 978-0-8153-5306-5 (hbk)
ISBN: 978-0-367-48771-3 (pbk)

Typeset in Bembo
by Apex CoVantage, LLC

To all interviewed dream characters and personifications of life issues, collectively called "emerging potentials," in appreciation for your guidance out of Plato's Cave and into the light.

Dream Sociomatrix

Author: Dillard
Dream Date: 8/27/01
Dream Name: Ken Wilber Dies
Smx Date: 8/27/01

Choosers: / *Chosen elements:*	Dream Self	Ken Wilber	Girlfriend	Car	Second Car	- Head on Crash	- Killed	*Very Upset	Other Driver								Character Raw Scores	Acceptance Axis Totals	Character Ambivalence
Dream Self	2	3	1			/3	/3	/3	/2								6/11	/5	M
Ken Wilber	3	3	3	1		/3	/3	2	/2								12/8	4	M
Girlfriend	2	3	2	1	/2	/3	/3	2	/2								10/10	0	D
Car	2	2	2	2/1	/3	/3	/2	2	/3								10/12	/2	H
Second Car						/3	/3	2	/2								2/8	/6	L
Other Driver				1		/3	/3	3	/3								4/9	/5	M
Dream Consciousness	3	3	3						3								12	12	
El. Raw Scores	12	14	11	4/1	1/6	/18	/17	1/3	/11										
El. Axis Totals	12	14	11	3	/5	/18	/17	8	/11										
EL Ambivalence																			

Scoring Key:

1 = like, 2 = like a lot, 3 = love; blank = indifference   "*" = feeling elements

/1 = dislike, /2 = dislike a lot, /3 = hate   * = complete acceptance   "--" = action elements

© 1985 Joseph Dillard. All Rights Reserved.

Contents

Preface

What is the relationship between the microcosm and the macrocosm? Are we predestined to be perpetually victimized by political, social, and natural forces outside of ourselves and beyond our control? Do we have the ability to alter such influences by our decisions, preferences, intention, and character? This is a fundamental question for humanity, and how we answer it largely determines our perspective toward ourselves and society, as well as what options for change we find realistic and available to us. Machiavelli, Hobbes, Skinner, Popper, and Darwin are proponents of the first view, while Lao Tzu, Socrates, Buddha, and Jesus were strong proponents for the latter. A third group believes that individuals of outstanding character, whom Confucius called the "Superior Man," can change society by first commanding and purifying their own characters.

Since Adam Smith, the first group, which we will call the "realists," has largely won the day and determined the fate of the world due to the subjugation of character to profit. As of 2016, even those members of the second group, who we shall call "idealists," and those in the third group, who we shall call "leaders," and who are dedicated to the advancement of the common good based on individual character, respect for international norms, and human rights, have largely succumbed to the pervasive and continuous incentive toward profit, as a survey of the ruling classes of contemporary democratic societies demonstrates. The most common solution, a massive social swing to an opposite pole of isolative collectivism, has been shown historically to bear the seeds of its own undoing.

Integral Deep Listening (IDL) recognizes these three as the exterior world, including the teachings of leaders, professionals, and gurus; the interior world, including the application of our judgment and common sense; and the internalization of healthy social norms for service based on conscience. To these three IDL adds a fourth, personal and social action directed by one's life compass, as defined by identification with a myriad of dream characters and the personifications of life issues, together referred to as "emerging potentials."

Dream Sociometry is a form of IDL that allows you to observe and understand the many patterns of preference that generate both your personality and your actions in the world. These interactive patterns not only reveal how and where you are both stuck and self-destructive; they lay out a path toward internal and intrasocial balance that brings personal order to interior experience and social order to relationships. If those interactive patterns depicted in the Dream Sociograms you create (and which are explained in the sequel to this text, *Understanding the Dream Sociogram*), are centered on your family, balance and order are likely to be observed to evolve away from social scripting, drama, and cognitive distortions and into a higher order of functioning based on priorities of life that are individualized as your "life compass." If those interactive patterns depicted in the Dream Sociograms you create are centered on your work or broader societal relationships, it is predicted that you will discover improved ways to maintain and assert your internal balance from the center of the hurricane of your social-cultural macrocosm.

Like meditation, IDL is a transpersonal integral life practice and yoga that anchors you in spaces that are in the world but not of it. Unlike meditation, IDL exposes where and how you are stuck and makes concrete recommendations about where you have the most leverage for growth, development, clarity, lucidity, waking up, and enlightenment. Dream Sociometry is a particularly intensive and effective version of IDL because it not only interviews a number of emerging potentials simultaneously; it compares their preferences with your own in order to provide you with unusual objectivity regarding the issues that concern you the most. This objectivity is both different from and more readily available than that found in meditation or society or gleaned from books or experts and is uniquely tailored to your own particular contexts. In some cases, particularly nightmares and repetitive dreams, such objectivity is enough to stop them once and for all. In other cases, particularly those that are maintained by multiple physical, psychological, and social-cultural factors, Dream Sociometry clarifies how you stay victimized while providing you with specific recommendations for moving ahead. Some recommendations will involve finding your own internal balance; others will involve taking concrete action in your relationships.

The examples of Dream Sociomatrices and Dream Sociograms found in this text are mostly those of the author, beginning in 1980, but reflect findings found with many clients in the decades since. *Dream Sociometry* was first written in 1985 as a text for students. I shared it with Stanley Krippner, then on the Board of the ARE Clinic in Phoenix, where I worked. He suggested a joint presentation at the yearly conference of the Association of the Study of Dreams and that I write an outline and first draft of a book on using dreaming for problem solving. That book, *Dreamworking: How to Use Your Dreams for Creative Problem Solving*, contained little to nothing on Dream Sociometry; it is much easier to teach through creating Dream Sociomatrices on one's own dreams or life issues so one can directly experience the process. This I did with students and clients in the late '80's and '90's and then with students at Southwest Institute for Healing Arts in Phoenix, where I taught from 1999 until 2007.

The delay in the publication of this material is due to a lack of professional peer interest, a lack of public response to the book that Krippner and I co-authored, which led to a general disinterest in anything but self-publishing, and the general complexity of organizing and presenting all the relevant supportive materials. It was only when I could finally get all examples referenced in both texts on line at www.integraldeeplistening.com and then refer to them in the text that it made sense to publish. It was only after I self-published both texts that I finally decided that the only way Dream Sociometry was likely to gain the attention of those counselors, coaches, and students of self-development who were likely to put it to serious use for personal transformation as well as to help others was if the texts were professionally published. I am very appreciative of both Daniela Simmons, PhD, psychodramatist and professor, who has applied Dream Sociometry with clients and in workshops, for referring me to Routledge, which is a respected publisher of noted works on psychodrama and psychology in general.

I have resisted the self-centered "all about me" navel-gazing implications of publishing a demonstration of the methodology based on my own rather trivial and insipid dreamlife. Finally, there was no good alternative, because while I had numerous examples of sociomatrices from students and clients, no one had worked up nearly as complete a series, which would be necessary if a community invested in this work were to collectively begin to create hypotheses of what we are seeing in these relationships, based on waking life issues, or series of dreams, something which I do in the second book in this series, *Understanding the Dream Sociogram*.

The particular example I use throughout the text, "Ken Wilber Dies," was chosen because it presents a short and concise treatment of a nightmare and is an example of working through a relationship with someone one respects immensely. While this example and indeed, most of this text deals with self-relationships (although I have never met or corresponded with Ken Wilber), it is important to remember that Dream Sociometry and IDL suspend assumptions about the ontology of interviewed elements: taking a phenomenological approach, it reduces them neither to self-aspects nor to shamanistic objective realities. Therefore, the reader is cautioned not to reduce this material to another form of "shadow" work. While it does indeed provide an extremely effective form of shadow work, the open-minded reader will recognize significant and common elements that have nothing to do with "shadow."

The field of Sociometry itself has evolved considerably since this text was written and the following methodology devised. Those who would like to compare it to further developments in the field are referred to Ann Hale's *Three Cyclical Models which enhance Consciousness of Interpersonal Connection* Published by International Sociometry Training Network and available at www.sociometry.net.

Dream Sociometry is an initial exploration, through character identification, of a dimension of life, the intrasocial, that belongs to everyone. Therefore, the author makes no claims of uniqueness or of ownership for Dream Sociometry. You are encouraged to take and use these concepts and methods as you so desire and to add your findings to the common heritage of humanity. The Dream Sociomatrices, Commentaries, and Dream Sociograms referred to in this text can be found under "Examples of Dream Sociometry" at www.integraldeeplistening.com.

October 11, 2017
Kähnsdorf, Brandenburg, Germany

Introduction

Dream Sociometry is an integral life practice and yoga based on the sociometric methodologies created by psychiatrist J. L. Moreno, creator of psychodrama and multiple experiential forms of psychotherapy. Dream Sociometry interviews multiple dream characters or elements in a waking circumstance, such as 9/11, or personal issues, such as cancer, a career change, or divorce.[1] This work has since been elaborated into a broader transmutational practice called "Integral Deep Listening" (IDL).[2]

Since Dream Sociometry was created in 1980, the world of research has witnessed a monumental turn toward inter-disciplinary studies, most powerfully and effectively represented by Ken Wilber's Integral AQAL. "AQAL," which stands for "all quadrants, stages, states, lines and types," summarizes a broad and deep cognitive multi-perspectival map that has generated multidisciplinary approaches to medicine, law, anthropology, physics, language, ecology, religion, spirituality, and, of course, psychology. This has in turn generated an enormously fertile depth of connectivity, not only among ideas, but among people on the cutting edge of a wide variety of professions.

This preface is intended to be an orientating overview of where the body of this text, which involves instruction in an injunctive methodology, lies in the context of first Wilber's AQAL and, more particularly, current integral thought, using the latter to also locate Dream Sociometry in the broad field of dream investigation.

Dream Sociometry is multi-perspectival

Dream Sociometry extends the concept of multi-perspectival in ways that initially may appear as outrageous, irreverent, profane, and irrelevant as Freud's Id-based theories of dreaming did to the Victorian English at the turn of the 20th century. Looking for meaning, much less transmutation, in spit or a blender and in their relationships to say, cartwheels or chimpanzees initially appears not only to be an exercise in self-centered projection, but a waste of time. However, integral has reaffirmed an ancient truth, that all points, all instances, all relationships, are worm-holes to, into, and, as Buzz Lightyear reminds us, even beyond the infinite, once we are armed with clear intention and a wise methodology. Clearly, a movement from a cognitive multi-perspectivalism to an experiential multi-perspectivalism, which is the purpose and function of *Dream Sociometry,* has to be undertaken from the outside in as well as from the inside out. As such, it is an enactment of the principle of non-exclusion, of *anekantavada.* Such an approach generates not only an introspective phenomenology in the upper right as a vehicle for practicing integral deep listening with intrasocial collectives, such as Sanghas of dream elements, in the lower left, cultural quadrant of holons, but also, through deep empathy, transmutes "Its" in the lower right, or social quadrant, of humanity, into "We" and "Us" and beyond that, into a non-dual "I" which enfolds both self and other as alternative framings of infinitely-faced Shivas at a Halloween party gone amuck.

Any child who has played "mommy" or "soldier" all the way up and through Dzogchen masters can use Dream Sociometry, or, its shortened forms, the IDL interviewing protocols and Dream Sociodrama, to get unstuck by first objectifying their blind spots and then marrying them with a life-transforming action plan.[3] Far broader than shadow work, and even the honored psychotherapeutic excursions of Gestalt, Dream Sociometry draws down fire from heaven and interweaves it with savory delights from the depths of Plato's Cave. Due to its integral nature, Dream Sociometry is a psychospiritual practice that can be applied to move forward on any developmental line and integrated into waking, meditative, dream, deep sleep, and mystical states. It is equally applicable to different styles, whether culturally scripted, gender-based, or professionally framed, because its basic structures and functions are as universal as dreaming, imagery, and empathy, as a core developmental unfolding.

We can view the current, ongoing and accelerating interdisciplinary thrust within and among multiple fields of knowledge as a breaking down of various cognitive dualisms. Traditionally, the work of deconstructing both cognitive and experiential dualisms has been left to the interior quadrant fields of mysticism, values, reframing interpretations and world views, and the generation of new paradigms. While interior quadrant approaches are essential, they are only half the picture, and Wilber has acknowledged same by identifying integral life practices in the major areas of body (nine practices), mind (six), spirit (eight), and shadow (seven) and the auxiliary areas of ethics (seven), sex (five), work (seven), emotions (six), and relationships (seven).[4]

Dream Sociometry extends this experiential emphasis within multi-perspectivalism into each of the four quadrants in order to deconstruct fundamental dualisms, including self vs. other, reality vs. fantasy, objective vs subjective, good vs. evil, secure vs. endangered, comfortable vs. stressed, life vs. death, sober vs. addicted, victim vs. persecutor/rescuer, loving/compassionate vs. selfish, conscience vs. immorality, Heaven vs. Earth, divine vs. profane, sacred vs. secular, God vs. self, Divine will vs. Sin, freedom vs. bondage, ultimate vs. conditioned truth, and clarity vs. delusion.[5] It does so in the interior individual (UL) quadrant of intention, private thoughts, and feelings by phenomenologically redefining the self as including but transcending the particular duality under consideration; in the interior collective (LL) quadrant of culture, value, interpretation, and world view, by identification with alternative perspectives, interpretations, and values that redefine our own perspective, interpretations, and values as including but transcending the duality; in the exterior individual (UR) quadrant of observable behavior by practicing a yoga, or integral life practice, that transcends and directs personal goal setting regarding both integral life practices and behavior in general; and in the exterior collective (LR) inter-objective quadrant of relationship, systems and society, by creating structures that are embodied, embedded, enactive, and extended.[6] This identification can be approached as a form of co-presence (Bhaskar, 2008), "the mutual in-dwelling of each being by all other beings, and their co-participation on the cosmic envelope: a holographic or nondual form of relatedness."[7] Instead of this co-presence generating a nondual self, it creates an open-ended, expansive, ability to dance without attachment from one identity to another.

Dream Sociometry is a dream yoga

As a yoga that involves dreams and dreaming, Dream Sociometry represents broader, more encompassing definitions of both "dream" and "yoga." It is neither a physical, *hatha* yoga, nor is it a *jnana. maya, bhakti, kundalini,* or *raja* yoga. It is instead a multi-perspectival transpersonal discipline, a behavior in the UR quadrant, that is meant to integrate not only other UR behaviors and integral life practices, but the realms and activities of the other three quadrants as well, using a trans-rational framework, that is, a methodology that is rational but which transcends rationality in significant ways. For example, when you interview a drunken octopus that is sitting on your head and quoting Einstein, although it appears preposterously irrational and pre-rational, you are hardly doing something that can be considered irrational, because it assumes a thoroughly rational methodology, but yields perspectives, beingness, and life processes that transcend and include both the prepersonal and the personal. Consequently, the relationships among both transcendent consciousness and social holons can be recognized, transformed and transmuted.[8] As such, it is also intended to provide context for directing and improving the quality of whatever other yogas and integral life practices one takes up through their organization and prioritization *via* triangulation.[9]

While state differences are real and significant enough from a psychologically geocentric perspective, these disappear from the perspectives of interviewed dream characters and the personifications of life issues, together referred to as "emerging potentials." Consequently, *Dream Sociometry* deconstructs the artificial state dualism between dreaming and waking life. Life itself does not appear to discriminate between dreaming and waking states, meaning that dreaming is as "real" as waking *while we are dreaming or lucid dreaming,* and waking is as illusory and delusionary as dreaming, when viewed from perspectives embedded in dream contexts. Dream Sociometry is a dream yoga in the sense that it an organizing and structuring discipline for all four quadrants in many states at most levels, from multiple perspectives that more accurately and inclusively personify the priorities not primarily of self, but rather, personifications of the priorities life itself.

Disidentification and identification, two processes that are fundamental to any intrasocial experiential multi-perspectivalism, are not only the polarities of manifested life, as evolution and involution, but are two faces of the "withdrawn" *virtual* described by Shaviro, Deleuze, and others, which enters into manifestation as emerging potentials.[10] We take this process of element identification, or inhabiting another perspective, for granted, because it is as familiar, profane, and immediate as breathing; it was the play-work of our childhood. However, as Wilber points out, disidentification-identification is the twin process by which we objectify our proximal self as distal selves, a process fundamental to growth on any and every developmental line. In addition, identification-disidentification is the developmental dialectic itself, in that identification is the stable, thesis "translative" phase, in which we spend most of our time, generating balance and homeostasis. Disidentification is the antithetical disrupter, yet capable of generating both transformation and transmutation if anticipated and approached with both creative enthusiasm and as upstream prevention. However, if antithesis is feared, rejected, ignored, or fought, as is often the case, then this disrupter generates what IDL terms "wake-up calls," first in the form of dream whispers, then repetitive dreams, then nightmares, then objectified waking dream-dramas, such as relationship issues, health problems, and "accidents." Obviously, diseases and life misfortunes are due to multiple factors; however, by welcoming antithesis through chosen disidentification and identification with personifications of such wake-up calls, Dream Sociometry can make higher-order synthesis more likely. This is a claim that you are not only invited to validate for yourself through the application of both cognitive and transpersonal epistemologies to Dream Sociometry, what Wilber calls the "eyes" of mind and spirit, but are *required* to do. For, as with any injunctive method, to become a peer, that is, someone whose feedback has validation, one has to follow the three injunctions of any empirical method: follow the instructions, do the experiments, and submit your results to peers in the method.

Bruce Alderman's grammatical philosophemes as applied to Dream Sociometry

Much of what follows in this preface is an application of an integral grammar of philosophy, as magnificently elaborated by Bruce Alderman in *Sophia Speaks,* to Dream Sociometry and to IDL in general.[11] While Wilber has stated that experience is essentially perspectival, Alderman notes that this approach prejudices a pronounal context, one of six basic grammatical philosophemes, all of which disclose fundamental and essential characteristics of ontology (being) and thereby clarify the uses and limits of epistemology (knowing). The others are nounal, adjectival, verbal or processual, adverbial, and prepositional. Each of these contextualize the identification-disidentification process in important, expressive ways. What the following framings, based on some of the newest and most promising thinking in integral, attempt to provide, is a pluralist onto-logical typology of dreaming in particular and more generally of imagery and, macrocosmically, of socio-cultural experience. From an integral mapping, each approach is true but partial; each is important in that it provides powerful, genuine, and useful understandings and approaches for advances in each of these three domains.

Pronoun-based approaches

A pronounal approach to Dream Sociometry, following thinkers such as Buber, Rosenszweig, Peirce, Habermas, and Wilber, views interviewed dream charac-ters and personifications of life issues as perspectives that are ontological reali-ties. Following Peirce, Wilber notes that nouns depend on a prior experience of the hearer with the object of the noun, while the pronouns "I," "You," "We," "It," "Its," and so forth are experientially immediate, meaning that they require no previous familiarity with their object. "Others," often perceived as "its" or even "heaps" or "artifacts," not worthy of holonic attribution, such as dirty socks or the asteroid belt are, with Dream Sociometry, not transformed, but transmuted into first "We" and "Us," as we respectfully and empathetically lis-ten, in a deep and integral way, to their values and perspectives, and then into "I," as we internalize, expand, and grow into identities that include yet tran-scends our own. As such, we are not simply disclosing an epistemology or way of knowing or of "looking at," but becoming a broader ontological presence, both expressed and withdrawn.

Each and every perspective is indeed partially a self-aspect, sub-personality, personal fantasy, or subjective delusion in that it is part of and party to our thoughts, feelings, and experience. Unless it is in some way dissociated, which is atypical, a dream crocodile or an imaginary turnip is both a self-aspect, yet unknown or recognized as such, and therefore generally perceived as an "it" in the lower right (LR) quadrant of systems and relationships. [12] For example, a thief in a nightmare is an aggressive "other;" he or she is an "it" in the LR quad-rant, which we understand to personify parts of ourselves with which we are in conflict. This is the understanding of "shadow" approaches based on Jung and advocated by Wilber. However, in addition to being a self-aspect, these perspec-tives can and do express significant degrees of autonomy, while providing world views that are not our own. As such, their authenticity is violated, through an act of reductionism, when we view them solely as self-aspects, "shadow," or frame them as denizens of a personal or collective unconscious.

Dream Sociometry demonstrates that the perceptual reality, as well as con-clusions derived from interviewing a vampire bat are as rational and useful as those derived from the same interviewed vampire bat viewing *you* as an artifact of *its* personal or collective unconscious, in shades of Chuang Tzu.[13] Throughout the interviewing process and even after identification, interviewed emerging potentials remain ontologically discrete, "other," and autonomous. As such, when Dream Sociometry is approached *via* a pronomial framing, "Its" in the LR become both "We's" and "Us" in the LL collective quadrant, while our sense of self in the UL quadrant expands to include both. We become them as much as they become us.

Application of recommendations in the UR through the integral life practice of dream yoga objectifies a phenomenological process, making it accountable to the global commons. This has far-ranging implications for integral ethics, which requires significantly increased grounding in the LR quadrant.[14] Therefore, pronomial framings of imaginative processes of all sorts, including conscious visual cognition, is powerful, effective, and useful, in that the ability to co-exist with multiple perspectives not only represents a higher-order tolerance of ambiguity, but both invites and incorporates multiple emerging potentials for problem-solving while avoiding epistemological reductionism.

Pronomial aspects of AQAL include its emphasis on perspectives. For example, AQAL is itself a form of cognitive multi-perspectivalism, a world view that incorporates and integrates multiple world views which are themselves perspectives. When AQAL approaches the four quadrants of holons as "Its," "We's," and "Is," it is framing holons from a pronomial perspective.

Types of dreamwork that take a primarily pronomial approach include all interpretive approaches in the tradition of ancient Egyptian dream interpretation, Artimidorus, Freud, and Jung, that is, that view dream contents as *symbols*, or representative perspectives, rather than as things in themselves, processes, or modes of being.

Such approaches emphasize transforming "Its" into "We" or "Us," and then to "I." This is observed in the assumption that "others" are psychological projections of self-aspects, to be re-owned through the taking of responsibility for their creation, beingness and meaning. This is essentially an interior collective quadrant focus because it emphasizes *interpretation*. It represents a psychologically geocentric world view in that these interpretations are made by the self, the locus of identity of the dreamer, whether asleep and dreaming or awake, and only secondarily by others.

Substantive, or noun-based, approaches

This same critique applies to nounal approaches, only the emphasis is more strongly placed on the ontological or substantial reality of interviewed elements. Cognitive linguistics views dream and imaginative images as radial or metaphorical extensions of discrete objects or experiences previously encountered in waking life.[15] In harmony with Object Oriented Ontology, which follows the philosophy of such thinkers as Democritus, Aristotle, Descartes,

Newton, Harmon, Bryant, and Wilber, objects of our awareness are ontologically real substances.[16] Similarly, Dream Sociometry notes that phenomenologically perceived entities, whether encountered during a dream, a lucid dream, or when interviewed, are bounded *things* as well as authentic, objectively experienced others, with the same unquestioned otherness as objects in the external reality you are experiencing at this moment.

For example, when you fully allow yourself to become a dragon with heartburn from a nightmare, whether during the dream or later, during an interview or later, during *sadhana*, its underlying reality provides an undeniably authentic context for its responses during the interview.

Nounal approaches to dreamwork are substantive and ontologically real. They involve encounter with entities that are intrinsically and fundamentally "other."

Nounal dreamwork approaches include shamanism, which is reflective of waking, concrete naïve realism that does not question the reality of that which presents itself as objectively "other." It also includes lucid dreaming, in which the lucid dreamer assumes that his or her experience is as real (or delusional) as waking, even though the dream is perceived to be a self-created reality. The thinking is something like this:

> While this porcupine is a self-created figment of my imagination, I have the power to turn it into a seductive soul mate and make passionate love to it. Therefore, I still experience it as an objective and real "other," only one that is self-generated and subject to my control.

Nounal approaches provide perhaps the best bridging between dreaming, whether non-lucid or lucid, and waking experience, in that both commonly assume naïve realism.

Mystical experience, whether in dreams, meditation or some other state are essentially nounal, because the experiencer returns quite convinced that they have not only experienced reality, but Reality, that is, not only personal truth, but collective, universal Truth that applies equally to everyone.

Near death experience is also primarily a nounal approach to experience for similar reasons.

Nounal approaches to Dream Sociometry view the being of each interviewed entity as individual, meaning that the universe is flooded with an unlimited number of authentic beings. However, this is not a shamanistic approach because shamanism assumes, in the concrete mode of naïve realism, that whatever is perceived in any state is alive in some other plane or dimension. While this is indeed a nounal approach to dream, mystical or other imagery, Dream Sociometry tables such assumptions in favor of simple phenomenalistic respect. Instead of presuming the reality or non-reality of the immediateness of this beingness, a form of projective mind-reading, we simply get out of the way as best we can and listen to its response to the questions in the interviewing protocol in a deeply respectful and integral way. Therefore, a nounal approach to Dream Sociometry approaches interviewed elements as authentic, real, and individual entities and holons, each with four quadrants, but does not impart a reality to them beyond their own remarks, while not taking these remarks at face value either. We are not dealing here with gods, but neither are we dealing with shadow. Instead, it is both/and, and, as with Nagarjuna and his tetralemma, the excluded middle. Doubt, analysis, and interpretation are tabled during the interview in order to give a priority to respectful listening. However, after the interview, interpretations are invited and re-employed.

Dream Sociometry does not make these interviewed elements into secondary substances, as Aristotle did and as followers of Freud and Jung do when they turn them into symbols. To do so deprives them of their substantiality by making their beingness dependent on some referent, rather than hearing, seeing, being and respecting each in its own right, for what and who it proclaims itself to be. Therefore, to take a nounal approach to Dream Sociometry is to not insist that these interviewed elements refer to anything or to associate them with any life issue or realm of personal meaning, at least not during the interview or later, when we return to a full identification with this or that element. However, at other times, when we return to our normal waking "I" as reference point, it is not only inevitable but helpful to create such references and generate such associations. It is a matter of *timing:* there is a time for full identification and phenomenological suspension of our assumptions, preferences, and expectations, and there is a time for using LL interpretations to incorporate what we have experienced into an expanded world view, an UL sense of self, UR behavior, and LR relationships.

Many metaphysical systems, ancient and modern, dismiss ordinary objects as unsophisticated and unworthy of philosophical attention and thereby generate a metaphysical dualism where none exists, is necessary, or helpful. This has been all the more so for dream elements and personifications of waking life issues, such as a fire that one might experience "burning" in their spinal prolapse. In this regard, we can borrow two concepts, Undermining and Overmining that Grahm Harman, the founder of modern object-oriented Philosophy, originated (Harman, 2011a). Undermining refers to one of two types of reductionism, the above-mentioned dismissing of dream and imaginary elements as unsophisticated and unworthy. Undermining makes the assumption that at least some categories of dream elements and waking fantasies are simply surface, superficial representations of some substantial referent reality "beneath" or "within." Viewing dream elements as symbols is an example of such undermining. An overmining reductionism commits the epistemological fallacy, that is, it contends that dream elements or personifications of life issues do not exist outside of perception, so that reality does not exist within these "others," but instead within the flow of experience itself.

Dream Sociometry avoids both of these approaches by first dropping such assumptions in a clear and simple phenomenological reduction and, secondly, by identifying with the "other" as completely as possible, in a way that might be reminiscent of possession by a Greek muse. This is somewhat of a threatening approach to many Westerners, who have been brought up to maintain self-control and individuality, while viewing the surrendering of self-control and the self as a regressive descent into decompensation and chaos. The methodology that you will learn here, when followed, demonstrates that myth for what it is: a scripted cultural bias that entombs the self in a rigid chrysalis from which it cannot escape and which slowly smothers it to death. The abandonment of these twin reductions allows Dream Sociometry to be viewed through the lens of "a democracy of objects," a concept that Harman and other object-oriented philosophers, such as Levi Bryant (2011a), Tim Morton (2011), and Ian Bogost (2012) embrace, and that Bryant coined (Bryant, 2011a).

In this regard, Dream Sociometry accepts the idea that we partially construct or "translate" the objects of our perception, say, when we interview a character and "become" it, either during the interview or later, while rejecting the idea that these elements are *nothing more* or could be anything other than human constructions. The reason why, besides obvious reductionism, is that it closes us off to negentropic aspects of life that are attempting to be born within us and through us. When we dismiss or minimize the ontology of an interviewed element, we are turning a presence that has sacred, kratophonic, and transcendent elements into something profane and secular before we have even given it a chance to disclose itself. Such dismissal discredits a basic principle of reciprocity: we are thereby so treating these elements in a way that we do not want to be treated ourselves.

Dream Sociometry also reflects ontological realism, the thesis that "objects are irreducible to our representations of them" (Bryant, 2011b). This principle seems obvious when elements are interviewed using Dream Sociometry. For example, the unique individuality and autonomy of a cyclops and peanut butter cup far transcends their relationship with each other, as depicted in the Dream Sociogram.[17] In that they often interpret the intention or meaning of their beingness in ways that we do not, it is manifestly obvious that they are not reducible to our representations of them.

While the application of principles of ontological realism to dreams and fantasies may seem quite strange and even bizarre to both philosophers and psychologists, it provides an important and significant validation of the autonomy and dignity of collectives in quadrants of both culture and society. It becomes impossible to dismiss the other as "Its" and thereby exploit or abuse them, or to dismiss the other as a figment of one's imagination and disregard or disrespect it. Both of these responses represent a failure of empathy, a fundamental therapeutic capacity that Dream Sociometry enlarges and entriches. Abstract philosophical principles are employed in tandem with a thanatomimetic methodology that generates a higher-order ethic in both the interior and exterior collective quadrants. In a very real sense, Dream Sociometry takes nounal philosophy to its necessary conclusion: the sacrilization of the delusional, illusory, and profane. However, it does not make the determination that an interviewed element is either an object or a thing, both or neither. A slab of butter or crayon can make that determination for itself, if it wants to.

Adjectival approaches

When a dream image is assumed to be a symbol, it often functions adjectivally, in that it personifies or represents qualities that modify what is the center of experience, generally, the substantial reality of the dreamer. For example, a storm cloud is assumed to personify the "stormy" temperament of the dreamer. In an adjectival ontology, such modifiers *are* reality; images do not stand for, represent, or modify some underlying substance or reality. The storminess is what is real, not some individual with some temperament.

When an adjectival, instead of a pronounal or nounal approach to interviewing elements is used, the result is rather Buddhist. Like the Buddhism of the *Dhammapada*, adjectival approaches note that things can only be known through their qualities – what they say and do, because their beingness is forever undisclosable. Because the beingness of a dream element cannot be directly experienced, its qualities are what are real. In the case of Buddhism, there is no self, or underlying ontological substance, only the five qualities, called *skandhas,* which interdependently co-originate to conjure up the delusion of a permanent self. However, against this position, it can be argued that the act of identification in Dream Sociometry involves becoming the beingness of the element itself, rather than simply knowing it indirectly through its qualities. Still, in so doing, while we encounter the fullness of beingness in the here and now, an objective assessment shows that this presence is *ad hoc,* flickering in and out of existence, based purely upon the attention that we give it. The temptation is therefore to reduce images to epistemological artifacts, holonic "heaps," products of our own "looking at" or knowing.

Dream Sociometry recognizes the legitimacy of this position by noting that it is not the form of this or that image that matters, but the intention behind, within, or beneath the qualities by which it is known. Is the ground toward which you are falling in a dream, hard, giving; does it transform into a feather bed, or does it disappear? If the quality itself is interviewed, rather than the ground itself, what does it have to say about itself?

An adjectival approach to dreamwork emphasizes the nature and interpretation of adjectival modifiers. Rather than focusing on the reality or non-reality of an element, or what perspective it takes, an adjectival approach attempts to enact or get to the meaning of "threatening," "confused," "ashamed," or "nauseated." Gestalt and psychodramatic approaches often take this approach, when they ask a client or auxiliary to take an "ashamed" position or act out the role of "threatening."

Verbal approaches

While a pronoun-based approach views being as perspective, a noun-based approach views being as substance, and an adjective-based approach views being as the appearance of its qualities, verbal-based approaches view being as process. Dreams are not about the dreamer but about whatever is going on in the dream or imagery – flying, walking, running, swimming. These actions, or lack of them, such as a dream rock sitting on a shore for eons, involve any dream element, not just the dreamer. Heraclitus, Plotinus, Hegel, Bergson, Whitehead, Hartshorne, Rescher, and Roy are some of the luminaries that have advocated the view that being is process. In this view, processes are ontologically more fundamental than substances or things because beings exist due to dynamic processes. For example, weather is a process, not a thing. Lightening, thunder, wind, rain, and snow are manifestations of underlying processes rather than real existent beings in their own right. According to Whitehead, what would be real about a dream buffalo is that it is an *actual occasion* which "prehends" its relation to other natural occasions – the other objects and elements in the dream, including the dreamer. Such an approach leans heavily, following Maturana and Luhmann, on an autopoietic, or self-generating process, but without their assumption that a self, object, or holon organizes or carries out that process.

The term IDL uses for dream elements and the personifications of waking life issues, "emerging potentials," resonates with a verbal or process-oriented approach to dreaming. Just as Whitehead's "actual occasions" relationally prehend the past and the future and thereby generate novel and emergent features in the process of actualization, so imagery appears to autopoietically self-create in interdependent relationship to its dream, mystical, drug-induced or waking context.[18] By so doing, it manifests in an emergent, or awakening form, possibilities, intentions, and potentials that are themselves processes. While creative emergence is transformational, when we take it forward by becoming the image in *sadhana*, it can be transmutational, in that what is emerging and potential can become actualized in the actual occasion we call ourselves. As we become what it is, who we are becomes identified with the emerging potentials inherent in those actual occasions that are being born not only into our awareness, but into our identity, our sense of who we are.[19]

Whitehead describes this process as *concrescence,* "the process by which entities become what they are through their relationships to other entities, while also contributing novelty through the unique ways in which those relations are integrated."[20] Concrescence is therefore an excellent way to understand how Dream Sociometry and IDL understand the autopoietic self-generation of imagery and their interdependent relationships to both other images and waking realities. The amazing variety of these relationships are elaborated in the sequel to *Dream Sociometry, Understanding the Dream Sociogram.* For Whitehead, and for verbally-based process approaches in general, nothing stands behind the connectivity of relationship. There is no one "doing" or "having" or "in" relationship. There is simply the co-arising of relationships among actual occasions. Again, this is a very Buddhist concept, in which *pratityasammupada,* or interdependent co-origination, replaces a self seeking salvation (as in Christianity), or the obedient self (as in Judaism and Islam), or a self seeking *ahimsa* (freedom) (as in Hinduism), or as a self seeking harmony and freedom from chaos (as in Chinese culture), as the central conception upon which its further premises and injunctions depend.

Dream Sociometry resembles in some regards Bonnitta Roy's processual thesis of direct perception as adequate participation. She writes,

> Because perspectives are shaped by "look for," as distinguished from the perception of "seeing," they too are part of the epistemological domain and are subject to persistent error, illusion and confusion and thus, persistently advance into higher and higher orders of complexity . . .[21]

While elements that are interviewed in Dream Sociometry are indeed perspectives shaped by "look for," when we become this or that perspective, say, a skunk, we shift from "look for" to "seeing," or direct phenomenological encounter and identification with that skunk. We are looking out at the world through its skunky eyes. By so doing, we are accessing a frame of information that we would normally not call our own and that most people would consider a perspective. This is the difference between a 2nd, or even 3rd-person perspective, and its transformation/transmutation into 1st person. We are becoming, or directly identifying, with that perspective, no longer "looking at," or objectively encountering it. Consequently, Dream Sociometry, and IDL interviewing in general, may qualify for what Roy would call "knowing as direct perception," or "knowing in the sense of Gnostic knowing." It is in this sense that identification with a perspective becomes transcendent of the ontological/epistemological dualism. Impermanence is the underlying reality; permanently existing things are constructs of processes that, given enough time, are shown to not be permanent or substantial at all. This is also a highly Buddhist view; it attributes the illusion of selves to the speed at which processes occur, creating the illusion of solidity and reality, as in a film; to the ability of the mind to recollect past experiences and therefore create causal chains of ownership; and to a lack of observational discrimination in the untrained mind.

Psychodrama and Gestalt therapy are approaches to dreamwork that emphasize a processual orientation, in that they are more interested in investigating the meaning and function of some dream or waking action in one's life rather than attributing it to someone or viewing it as a perspective. A psychodramatist might have the subject and auxiliaries run around the room to explore the meaning of "running," or they might give voice to "burning," "digesting," "drinking," or "smoking." What then becomes important in the understanding of the dream or life issue is the meaning of some action, not its attribution or the discovery of some one "right" meaning.

Adverbial approaches

In an adverbial approach to Dream Sociometry and the therapeutic identification with imagery in general, like adjectival approaches, images symbolically or metaphorically represent, stand in for, depict, or modify an underlying reality, such as a bodhisattva, ghost, or larvae, as these can be seen as the embodiment of a mode of becoming. When we become them we are pulled into their own distinct field of becoming: Maitreya is going to take us places that Padmasambhava or Avalokitesvara will not; a ghost will take you places an Uber driver will not; a larvae will have you experience a unique unfolding, depending on whether you embody the process of becoming a fly or food for SkyNet in the Matrix.

Adverbial approaches explore the various ways that images function as processes. Examples of such relational modes, according to Heidegger, include space, world, self, others, possibility, matter, function, meaning, and time. For Whitehead, such relational modes include color, form, pattern, number, space, time, and gravity, and these describe, adverbially, *how* actual occasions emerge prehensively into existence. From an adverbial standpoint, dream images, which are processes, not substances or perspectives, are actualizing themselves through this or that adverbial pathway or "modal expression." Is its spatial relationship what is emphasized by a waterfall when interviewed, or is it its size, function, its meaning, or *when* its water crashes into the pool below in the dream? All these are adverbial modes of expression, and any interviewed element is going to emphasize some more than others, and these will be vital to understanding its autopoietic self-generation in terms of process, or what it does in the dream or life context that it embodied.

Where, as in the case of image as adjective, the underlying reality "symbolized" is a substance, in the case of image as adverb, the underlying reality "symbolized" is a process, whether some other modifier, such as an adjective, another adverb, or a verb itself, such as the growing into some embodiment.[22] Instead of asserting its reality apart from what it modifies, as adjectival approaches do when they depict the way that the dreamer feels and what she thinks when she is crying as being the reality, adverbial approaches do not generally claim to replace or substitute for the underlying reality of the process at hand. Crying itself is the reality. Instead, they complement or add descriptive depth to what is basically a verbal approach to understanding what is going on when we dream and when we identify with some metal image.

An adverbial approach to dreamwork will emphasize the way in which this or that element embodies some process of becoming. Is it being done out of some role in the Drama Triangle? Is the element speaking or acting in a persecuting, victimized, or rescuing manner? Is becoming being fought, welcomed, or ignored?

Eastern approaches that see life as a dream can be viewed as adverbial, in that all states are not only processes, but experiential modes, lacking any intrinsic reality. The underlying "reality" not only lacks *bhava*, "own being"; it is delusional. Dreaming is the mode of becoming that modifies the action of living. However, note that Eastern approaches are not consistent in this stance in the same way that post-modernism is, in that both Vedanta and Madhyamika take refuge in fundamental dualisms of relative and absolute truths, or realms that are finally substantive and nounal.

Whether images as complementing modes of verbal processes are conceived in pluralistic (Heidegger), monistic (Spinoza), or non-dual framings (Whitehead, Tibetan Buddhist Dzogchen, or Kashmiri Shaivism), they all emphasize the importance of how an image manifests itself in relationship to other things, which are all equally substantial or insubstantial images, depending on which position you take. Indeed, these various approaches apply equally to "real" and "imaginary" "things" or "beings," as noted by Rescher (1996), Object Oriented Ontology, and Actor Network Theory, as described by Harman in *The Prince of Networks* (2009).

Interestingly, Buddhism and Hinduism are not consistent in their application of this perspective to dreaming. They regress to an essentially nounal psychological geocentrism, in which the self does the interpretation of experiences that are either sacred and real or profane and illusory.

Prepositional approaches

A common thread in all these approaches is the question, "Is there something beneath, behind or within images that creates them or do they create themselves?" Is their essence derivative of an underlying substantial ontology or are surfaces the ontology itself? Notice that the key words in these questions, "beneath," "behind," "within," and "underlying" are *prepositions*: they are not things or objects in themselves but describe types of relationships. These are *bridging* concepts, that connect one something with another. When you focus on relationship or bridge itself, as the source of meaning, substance and being, you create a prepositional ontology. Thinkers who have done so include Latour, Souriau, Nancy, Serres, and Sloterdijk, indicating the post-modern and contemporary arising of this latest approach to the framing of reality.

Prepositions may modify both nouns and verbs, functioning as both adjectives and adverbs, while being neither. Consequently, they are perhaps the most encompassing or multi-perspectival (what Latour calls "plurimodal") of the various approaches to imagery that have preoccupied humanity to this point. They do not attempt to restrict humanity to the metaphysical deadlock of one mode of being or another. However, they are also the most abstract.

From the perspective of IDL, prepositional approaches attempt to transcend dualities by emphasizing the underlying reality of interdependent relationship. For example, in a dream where you are attacked by a man with a knife, there is an obvious duality. However, when you interview the knife, the duality is likely to disappear, replaced by an awareness of an interdependent, co-created relationship, what Nancy (2000) refers to as the "with" of "being singular plural." By emphasizing "with," Nancy is indicating the primacy of equivalency of relationship among beingness as individually or collectively constructed. It becomes obvious that the man, the knife and "you" are not the underlying realities, objects or functions of the drama, but rather modes depicting multi-perspectival relationships, the fabric of which can be expressed by various means, including the interdependent constellations explored in Dream Sociograms. Note that exactly the same processes of encounter apply to say, a terrorist attacking a group of people in waking life; life itself makes no differentiation, and the same "with," that is, "being singular plural," applies to it as well, and, likewise, a similar "coessentiality" can be depicted interdependently in a Dream Sociogram.

From a prepositional framing, "subjects and verbs are derivative and verbs must follow the flows that prepositions make available."[23] The result for Dream Sociometry is that relationship and interaction is primary, and these are determined by subtle, inferred connective intentionalities that point out a type of relationship, but then leave it to specific dream elements and waking images and processes in both realms to enact. Such an approach doesn't care who or what character is represented in waking life or dreaming, or even what they are doing; what matters are the underlying intentions that are depicted by arbitrary relationships and actions. Depicted elements are arbitrary in that other relationships, characters, and actions could make the same point just as well. Dream Sociometry can be viewed as a highly prepositional approach in that its Dream Sociograms emphasize the depiction of relationships and the intentionalities that they personify. For example, are characters, actions, and feelings in opposition or agreement? Is the intention of the group united in the embodiment of growth, or do intrasocial dynamics depict antithetical relationships?

Prepositional windows on reality therefore force a non-dualistic, relational perception of experience, moving non-dualism from the realm of the mystical and transpersonal into the domain of mundane, everyday experience. This breaks down the classical distinction between "sacred" and "profane," "meaningful" and "meaningless" "day residue" imagery.

While Nancy and the other prepositionalist philosophers make a case for relational non-dualism on a cognitive level, Dream Sociometry takes a phenomenalistic and experiential, multi-perspectival approach that takes into account not only approaches that are biased toward perspectives, such as pronounal ones, but which attempt to honor and include the contributions of each of these various grammatically based approaches to understanding reality. We are invited to think of all four quadrants at once instead of dividing reality into individual and collective ontologies that occupy interior or exterior spaces in possessive or non-possessive ways.[24]

As I write this in the fall of 2017, almost 40 years after developing Dream Sociometry, in the spectacular lake-filled countryside of Brandenburg in northeastern Germany, as the fall equinox once again approaches, I observe a rising desire to take the vast cognitive multi-perspectival map of integral and ground it experientially in ways that affirm life in the world, in order to address the underlying issues of selfishness, greed, inequality, and discrimination that continue to largely rule both individuals and humanity as a whole. Both metanoia, or transformation, as the changing of suffering into transcendence, and transmutation are not only possible, but increasingly recognized to be essential, if we are to address the multiple causes of the equally multiple catastrophes that humanity has visited upon itself and the planet. A hymn familiar in New Age circles famously begins, "Let there be peace on Earth and let it begin with me." The intention is to affirm personal responsibility for recognizing and ameliorating the interior, or microcosmic, etiological factors that are projected outward onto the other in forms of life problems, interpersonal conflicts, economic exploitation, discrimination, and the deconstruction of living systems. However, personal responsibility can be taken too far; reality creates us as much as we create it. The macrocosm, in the form of issues of public policy, terraforming, governance, public health, and many other issues, is equally important and demand equal emphasis. Dream Sociometry, as a collective approach to owning the macrocosm by expanding our self-definition to encompass it, embraces an integral methodological pluralism not simply as a cognitive mapping, but as a personally enacted commitment to humanity and life itself.

Notes

1 An example of Dream Sociometry with 9/11 as well as examples with dreams and life issues are found *at* IntegralDeepListening.Com, "Examples."
2 See *Dream Yoga.Com* and ***IntegralDeepListening.Com***.
3 For examples of the protocols and Dream Sociodrama see http://www.integraldeeplistening. com/questionnaires/ Many examples of single element interviews, both of dreams and life issues, are available at the **blog** of IntegralDeepListening.Com.
4 Wilber, K., Patten, T., Leonard, A., & Morelli, M. (2008). *Integral Life Practice: A 21st-Century Blueprint for Physical Health, Emotional Balance, Mental Clarity and Spiritual Awakening.*
5 An explanation of how Dream Sociometry and more broadly, IDL deconstruct these dualities is in Dillard, J. *Healing Integral, Pt 2: Transformations for the Future*, pp. 27–36.
6 Thompson, Evan. (2015b). "*Context matters*: Steps to an embodied cognitive science of mindfulness." UC Davis Center for Mind and Brain research summit "Perspectives on Mindfulness: the Complex Role of Scientific Research."
7 Alderman, B., *Integral in-Dwelling*, p. 9.
8 For example, see Lex Neale's AQAL Cube.
9 Dillard, J. (2015). *Waking Up*, Deep Listening Press, Berlin. Also: http://integraldeeplistening. com/triangulation-a-superior-approach-to-problem-solving/
10 (Shaviro, 2010)
11 Alderman, B. *Sophia Speaks: An Integral Grammar of Philosophy*. Alderman_ITC2013.pdf
12 In Wilber's integral theory, humans and entities, including dream characters, are "holons," consisting of four major "quadrants." These are the interior individual upper left (UL) phenomenological quadrant of largely undisclosed feelings, thoughts, and intentions; the interior collective lower left (LL) inter-subjective quadrant of values, interpretations, world views and culture; the exterior individual upper right (UR) behavioral quadrant of observable and measurable structures and processes; and the exterior collective lower right (LR) inter-objective quadrant of interaction, systems, and society..

13 "I dreamed I was a butterfly, flitting around in the sky; then I awoke. Now I wonder: Am I a man who dreamt of being a butterfly or am I a butterfly dreaming I am a man?" *Zhuangzi.*
14 See Dillard, J. (2017). *Healing Integral.* Berlin: Deep Listening Press.
15 (Lakoff & Johnson, 1999)
16 (Robinson, 2004; Bryant, 2011a; Harman, 2011c)
17 The Dream Sociogram provides a visual representation of the patterns of interdependent co-arising of intrasocial collectives, whether originating in dreams, life issues, mystical states, or drug trips. Examples are associated with the Dream Sociomatrices noted above, and an exegesis of their patterns of relationship is a topic of *Understanding the Dream Sociogram.*
18 Emergence and autopoiesis are two of five generative processes that Roy and Trudel (2011) have identified. The other three are construction, development, and evolution.
19 This is not unlike the Tibetan Buddhist practice of yidam, discussed by Bezin, A., in *What Is the Difference Between Visualizing Ourselves as a Buddhist Deity and a Deluded Person Imagining They Are Mickey Mouse?* and answered in Dillard, J., *Tibetan Yoga and Integral Deep Listening.*
20 Alderman, B. *Sophia Speaks*, p. 45.
21 Roy, B. *Gnostic Revival.*
22 "Smbolized" is placed in quotes to indicate that this is an assumption and projection by waking identity that is not typically made by interviewed elements.
23 Alderman, B. *Sophia Speaks*, p. 70.
24 "Possessive and non-possessive" is a reference to Lex Neale's third dimension in his AQAL Cube expansion of holons.

Bibliography

Alderman, B. (2012). Opening space for translineage practice: Some ontological speculations. *Journal of Integral Theory and Practice*, 7(2), 49–71.
Bhaskar, R. (2008). *A realist theory of science.* New York: Routledge.
Bogost, I. (2012). *Alien phenomenology, or what it's like to be a thing.* Minneapolis, MN: The University of Minnesota Press.
Bohm, D. (1980). *Wholeness and the implicate order.* New York: Routledge.
Browne, CG. (1951) *Study of executive leadership in business.* Psycnet.apa.org/record71951-07151-001
Bryant, L. (2008). *Correlationism and the fate of philosophy.* Retrieved from http://larvalsubjects.wordpress.com/2008/06/13/correlationism-and-the-fate-of-philosophy/
Bryant, L. (2010a, June 27). *Whitehead's prehensions and onticology.* Retrieved from http://larvalsubjects.wordpress.com/2010/06/27/whiteheads-prehensions-and-onticology/
Bryant, L. (2010b, July 1). *Even more Vitale: Translations, perspectives, and truth.* Retrieved from http://larvalsubjects.wordpress.com/2010/07/01/even-more-vitale-translations-perspectives-and-truth/
Bryant, L. (2011a). *The democracy of objects.* Ann Arbor, MI: MPublishing.
Bryant, L. (2011b, April 12). *OOO realism and epistemology.* Retrieved from http://larvalsubjects.wordpress.com/2011/04/12/ooo-realism-and-epistemology/
Bryant, L. (2011c). The ontic principle: Outline of an object-oriented philosophy. In L. Bryant, N. Srnicek, & G. Harman (Eds.), *The speculative turn: Continental materialism and realism.* Melbourne, Australia: re.press. 81.
Bryant, L. (2011d, February 2). *The time of the object: Toward the ontological grounds of withdrawal.* Retrieved from http://larvalsubjects.files.wordpress.com/2010/12/timeofobject-10- tex-1.pdf

Bryant, L. (2012, March 14). *Alethetics*. Retrieved from http://larvalsubjects.wordpress.com/2012/03/14/alethetics/

Harman, G. (2005). *Guerilla metaphysics: Phenomenology and the carpentry of things*. Chicago: Open Court.

Harman, G. (2009). *Prince of networks: Bruno Latour and metaphysics*. Melbourne, Australia: Re.Press.

Harman, G. (2011a). *The quadruple object.* Winchester, UK: Zero Books.

Harman, G. (2011b). On the undermining of objects: Grant, Bruno, and radical philosophy. In L. Bryant, N. Srnicek, & G. Harman (Eds.), *The speculative turn: Continental materialism and realism*. Melbourne, Australia: re.press.

Harman, G. (2011c). Response to Shaviro. In L. Bryant, N. Srnicek, & G. Harman (Eds.), *The speculative turn: Continental materialism and realism*. Melbourne, Australia: re.press.

Harman, G. (2011d). The road to objects. *Continent, 1*(3), 171–179.

Hartshorne, C. (1979). Whitehead's revolutionary concept of prehension. *International Philosophical Quarterly, 19*(3), 253–263.

Hauser, M. D., Chomsky, N., & Fitch, T. W. (2002). The faculty of language: What is it, who has it, and how did it evolve? *Science, 298*(5598), 1569–1579.

Heidegger, M. (1962). *Being and time*. (J. MacQuarrie & E. Robinson, Trans.). New York: HarperCollins Publishers.

Lakoff, G., & Johnson, M. (1999). *Philosophy in the flesh*. NY: Basic Books.

Latour, B. (2011). Reflections on Etienne Souriau's Les differents modes d'existence. (S. Muecke, Trans.). In L. Bryant, N. Srnicek, & G. Harman (Eds.), *The speculative turn: Continental materialism and realism*. Melbourne, Australia: re.press.

Morton, T. (2011). Here comes everything: The promise of object-oriented ontology. *Qui parle, 19*(2), 163-190.

Nancy, J. (2000). *Being singular plural*. (R.D. Richardson & A.E. O'Byrne, Trans.). Stanford, CA: Stanford Unity Press.

Rescher, N. (1996). *Process metaphysics: An introduction to process philosophy*. Albany, NY: State University of New York Press.

Robinson, H. (2004). Substance. In E.N. Zalta (Ed.), *The Stanford encyclopedia of philosophy*. (Winter 2009 Ed.). Retrieved from http://plato.stanford.edu/archives/win2009/entries/substance/.

Rogers, CG., (1946) *Significant aspects of client-centered therapy.* Chicago: Univ. of Chicago.

Roy, B. (2006). A process model of integral theory. *Integral Review, 3*, 118–152. Retrieved March 1, 2012, from http://integral-review.org/back_issues/backissue3/index.htm, 84.

Roy, B. (2010, July). *AQAL 2210: A tentative cartology of the future, or how do we get from AQAL to a-perspectival?* Paper presented at the biannual Integral Theory Conference, Pleasant Hill, CA. Retrieved from http://integraltheoryconference.org/sites/default/files/itc-2010-papers/Roy_ITC%202010.doc.pdf

Roy, B., & Trudel, J. (2011, August). Leading the 21st century: The conception-aware, object-oriented organization. *Integral Leadership Review*. Retrieved February 27, 2012, from http://integralleadershipreview.com/3199-leading-the-21stcentury-the-conception-aware-object- orientedorganization

Shaviro, S. (2009). *Without criteria: Kant, Whitehead, Deleuze, and aesthetics*. Cambridge, MA: The MIT Press.

Shaviro, S. (2010, August 1). *Whitehead vs. Spinoza & Deleuze on the virtual*. Retrieved from **www.shaviro.com/Blog/?p=909**

Van Zelst., (1952) *Sociometrically selected work teams increase production*. Personnel Psychology. Vol.5, Issue 3. Sept. 1952.

Varela, F. J. (2000). Steps to a science of inter-being: Unfolding the dharma implicit in modern cognitive science. In G. Watson, S. Batchelor, & G. Claxton (Eds.), *The psychology of awakening: Buddhism, science, and our day-to-day lives* (pp. 71–89). York Beach, ME: Samuel Weiser, Inc.

Whitehead, A. N. (1967). *Adventures of ideas*. New York: The Free Press.

Whitehead, A. N. (1978). *Process and reality*. New York: The Free Press.

Chapter I

What is Dream Sociometry?

A multi-perspectival path to the transpersonal

Dream Sociometry is an in-depth character and life issue interviewing protocol that is one aspect of Integral Deep Listening (IDL). IDL is itself a form of dream yoga, or a path to awakening from the dreamlike nature of reality, asleep or awake. IDL does not claim that life is a dream, only that it shares with dreaming the same common delusion that while asleep and dreaming one is awake. It also shares with dreaming the ability to wake up, or move into lucidity and out of the delusion, that occurs with lucid dreaming. Dream Sociometry is *multiperspectival* because it asks you to take a variety of different world views or orientations that are invested in individual dreams and life dramas. It is *transpersonal* because it provides both temporary state and permanent stage access to holons that transcend, yet include, both rational/personal and belief/preference-based prepersonal levels of development.

The Dream Sociomatrix is a grid-based structure that is used to obtain interviewed character preferences, tabulate them, and provide numerical data which are tabulated and plotted on a Dream Sociogram. It is accompanied by elaborative remarks which make up the various Commentaries. The Dream Sociomatrix for the dream *Ken Wilber Dies* is an example of such a grid, recording the likes and dislikes of interviewed characters toward each listed element (interviewed character, action, or emotion) in the dream. The Dream Sociogram is a pictorial representation of the patterns of preferences among choosing characters and chosen characters, actions, and emotions. These components of Dream Sociometry provide many benefits, as we shall note below. Most fundamentally, the process is transpersonal, in that it is designed to cultivate both witnessing and witnessing of the witness, as well as multi-perspectivalism in service to the deconstruction of identification with any and all identities or definitions of self.

An integral life practice

Interviewing is one of five major components of IDL. The first three emphasize reducing the filters that keep you stuck in dreamlike delusion: recognizing and

altering your life scripting, opting out of the Drama Triangle and recognizing and changing your emotional, logical and perceptual cognitive distortions.
The remaining two are transpersonal: developing highly empathetic multi-
perspectivalism with IDL interviewing, and meditation, including naming and
pranayama. These five are together components of a sophisticated integral life
practice that sets life priorities in consultation with your life compass. Your life
compass is not to be confused with intuition, "soul," conscience, divine will, a
"still small voice," dharma, karma, or predestination. It is represented in IDL
by the consensual perspectives of characters and life issues, together referred
to as "emerging potentials," that you become and interview. IDL teaches you
to deeply listen to the diamond wisdom of deathless emerging potentials that
personify the priorities of life.

"Emerging potentials" refers to interviewed perspectives with which you
identify, whether during an interview or sometime thereafter: for instance,
when you are meditating, at work, or arguing with your partner. These perspectives may be derived from elements with which you identify or the personifications of life issues that are important to you. They may also be mythological,
literary, historical, or religious in origin. They are neither self-aspects nor external realities, but rather contain important, irreducible aspects of both, in that
they are undoubtedly both self-creations and autonomous, capable of expressing great independence from your assumptions, preferences and world view.
Emerging potentials cannot be categorized as unconscious, subconscious or
superconscious, spiritual or mundane, prepersonal, personal or transpersonal,
irrational, rational, or arational or trans-rational. They are not symbols, nor are
they archetypes.

Rather than finding your growth chronically held hostage by your daily dramas, scripting, addictions, and fixations, IDL progressively expands your ability
to witness the endless parade of hopes, thoughts, feelings, and relationships that
fill your life. This is a concrete type of witnessing, in that it produces practical
and personalized recommendations for getting unstuck and moving your reality into deeper alignment with the priorities of life.

The art of deeply listening to the priorities of your life compass is intrinsically healing, providing the integration and balancing of your various life
roles. As you experience the harmony, wisdom, and acceptance of life as it
uniquely expresses itself through you, you can then move forward in inner
consensus rather than as a dictatorial ego attempting to force compliance
from repressed, ignored, and discounted feelings, preferences, and desires.
This allows you to progress on your life's journey as a whole rather than as
a fragmented being. Instead of leaving important parts of yourself behind
as dead weight, slowing or stopping your development, you welcome them
into an expanded definition of who you are. Instead of living within your
self definitions, you open yourself to broader framings represented by interviewed emerging potentials. As your identity expands, a partnership is forged
between you and your intrasocial community, leading you to first become

one with your life compass, then with life itself, as you move your life experience into transpersonal perspectives.

Your "intrasocial community" is comprised of 1) self-aspects, such as your preferences and addictions, 2) others, including your exterior or disowned reality, to the extent that what you know of other people, places, or objects is a projection of your own experience, values, and meanings, and 3) interviewed emerging potentials, which combine elements of both self and other but which cannot be reduced to either. Together, these serve as wake-up calls that, when deeply listened to, both expand and thin your sense of self.

Dream Sociometry is the foundational methodology that IDL uses to accomplish waking up, clarity, lucidity, and progressive enlightenment. However, in practice, IDL usually relies on interviews of individual elements, due to its relative simplicity. Dream Sociometry is used as both a research tool and as a way for students to become thoroughly grounded in the principles that underlie the various individual element interviewing protocols.[1] Its object is to provide a structure by which your life compass can alchemically transform the secular and mundane clay of your life into the precious gold of the sacred. It does so through two processes: unearthing and resolving all sorts of conflicts that block your further development and shifting your identity from yourself to identification with life's perspectives and agendas, and by creating space in which expanded, more inclusive awareness can be born.[2] Dream Sociometry is a tool that allows you to not only step back and watch yourself go by, but to deeply listen to and learn from emerging potentials that not only support your development but that also oppose you and thereby slow your development. You will also find yourself amazed by the perspectives on your life provided by interviewed emerging potentials, whether angelic messengers or toilet brushes, that are not stuck in the same ruts that currently bog down your progress. As you merge with perspectives that include, yet transcend, your own, you assimilate their fearlessness and objectivity, thereby diffusing and broadening your identity.

While Dream Sociometry can be used effectively for such secular purposes as finding a job, a mate, or creative problem solving in groups or industry, when it is used to become one with life itself, it becomes a form of yoga. It also serves as a yoga when secular goals, such as career and relationship success, are approached from the context of transpersonal purposes, such as living one's life more in harmony with the priorities of one's life compass.[3]

Dream Sociometry involves the eliciting of the preferences of interviewed dream characters or personifications of life issues important to you along with the collection of explanations of their preferences, called *elaborations*. Other approaches to interviewing taught by IDL include the dream and life issue protocols used for interviewing individual perspectives and *DreamQuest!*, a character interviewing game. Dream Sociometry is most often approached as a self-directed approach, although it can be used with others: for example, when a couple or work group creates sociomatrices on the same, commonly shared issue, controversy, conflict, or work problem. By applying Dream Sociometry to a series of your own dreams waking life "dreams" and nightmares, you can familiarize yourself with the underlying principles of IDL interviewing.

Most students of IDL will already be familiar with the single-character interviewing protocol, which questions individual elements and other emerging potentials, such as emotions or characters taken from actual waking life events. Dream Sociometry is the foundation for the single-character interviewing protocol. I only reluctantly developed that methodology after years of largely unsuccessful efforts to make Dream Sociometry more accessible to a broader number of people. Dream Sociometry takes longer and provides much more information than most people want or can use. Therefore, for years, I regarded it primarily as a research tool. It was only after a number of years of including Dream Sociometry in the IDL Practitioner training program and listening to the positive feedback of students who already had a strong foundation in the single character interviewing protocols that I returned to my original belief, that Dream Sociometry had important practical and not just research-based applications.

The dream and life issue interviewing protocols contain many of the core principles of Dream Sociometry in various forms, but without the depth that comes from interviewing multiple perspectives and without the advantage of the visual representation of intrasocial dynamics provided by the Dream Sociogram. In addition to being foundational, Dream Sociometry is extremely versatile, providing a very extensive and thorough approach to transpersonal development that can be pursued in isolation by monks, prisoners, introverts, or the highly analytical, or in couples and groups for relationship, family, work, and socio-cultural applications. Dream Sociometry can be an important component of a transpersonal *discipline*, which is what a yoga is meant to be. The two-plus hours that are spent on a dream with Dream Sociometry provide a treasure trove of assistance in growth, healing, and life balancing.

A third reason to become familiar with Dream Sociometry is to give depth to your interviewing of emerging potentials and therefore speed your development. Understanding Dream Sociometry explains the genesis for many of the questions used in the IDL dream and life issue protocols, examples of which you will find in the appendices. The questions they contain are largely drawn from those in the various Dream Sociometric elaborations discussed below. Creating Dream Sociometrices deepens both confidence and understanding of why each particular question is asked. Dream Sociometry also generates opportunities to cultivate your experience of the pure witness and subject permanence through identification with that consciousness which creates dreams and, by analogy, creates all form.[4] This experience is of immense importance for those desiring either to find or integrate non-dual awareness into their meditative or daily life. Finally, for those of you who wish to become teachers of IDL, or life coaches, personal familiarity with Dream Sociometry is a requirement, since you must understand it in order to be able to teach it to others. Learning

Dream Sociometry will add great depth of understanding and application to your work with the single-character interviewing protocols.

In the Dream Sociometric method, as in the single-character interviewing protocol process, you first identify three life issues that are of current concern to you. You then imagine that you are various interviewed characters in your recalled dream or waking life experience and write down how you feel about yourself, the dreamer, and what is going on in your dream.[5] The preferences of interviewed elements are given numerical values. These are: love = +3; like a lot = +2; like = +1; don't care = 0; dislike = −1; dislike a lot = −2; hate = −3; and transcending all preferences = *.[6] These numerical values are noted in a grid-like data collection form called a *Dream Sociomatrix*. It provides a way to step back and look objectively at what aspects of your larger identity have to say to you about why you have the issues you are dealing with now in your life and what you need to do about them, from their perspective.

The Dream Sociomatrix provides for the orderly tabulation and evaluation of the preferences expressed by different interviewed characters. The expression of these preferences usually elicits thoughts and feelings. These are written as elaborations in a section following the Dream Sociomatrix, called the *Sociomatrix Commentary*. Information from all these processes does much more than provide insight into the dream or waking life issue; it is used to integrate your waking and dream lives, which is a powerful support for both waking up and the development of clear consciousness. To this end, there follows a special set of directions for using character recommendations to resolve waking life issues you have identitied. These elaborations include a *Dream Commentary*, in which emerging potentials generate an integrative revision of the dream, called a *dreamage*. It also includes a *Waking Commentary*, in which characters recommend changes in your waking life. An *Action Plan* is created that specifies situations in which it will be beneficial for you to imagine you are this or that character in your waking life. Information from this process can also be used to create and understand the *Dream Sociogram*, which depicts patterns of intrasocial interaction.

A phenomenalistic approach to dream interpretation

While the reader will discover many similarities to other approaches to dreamwork, most of those similarities are superficial. Dream Sociometry differs in significant ways from the Gestalt role-play of Fritz Perls, the emphasis on symbolic interpretation of Freud, Jung, and Cayce the projective group processes of Montague Ullman or the Voice Dialogue methodologies of the Stones. Dream Sociometry shares with Perl's Gestalt common phenomenalistic roots in Jacob Moreno's sociometric and psychodramatic theories and methods. It may also remind students of comparative dreamwork methods of the phenomenological approach taken by Walter Bonime, but I have no background and scant familiarity with his work, which I nevertheless respect for its emphasis on the laying aside of reality claims.

Dream Sociometry draws upon early subjective methods in psychology that place emphasis on self-direction through the development of those introspective skills that provide a measure of objectivity toward oneself. It strives to be integrative, meaning that it respects and attempts to take into account many of the important distinctions set forth in the integral psychology of Ken Wilber, in that it is mindful of the level and line of interviewed perspectives, all four holon quadrants, the stage of development of the self and the implications of findings for waking, dreaming, deep sleep, and meditative experience.[7]

"Phenomenalistic" approaches to life suspend reality claims. In IDL, interviewed perspectives are not approached initially as subjective, self-created symbols or self-aspects or as real beings from some other dimension, but as beings possessing the same degree of reality that you do. If you are real, they are real as well, because they are both projections and reflections of your consciousness. If you are a figment of your own imagination, they are figments as well. While their ontology is indeterminate, their axiology or value is presumed to be due respect until proven otherwise, just as yours is. This is because you and all beings are interdependently co-created and mirror or reflect one another. Therefore, all are due respect until proven otherwise. While this is not a phenomenalistically neutral position, respect is a necessary precondition, because to discount the value of any perspective is to discount the value of those identities that they personify or represent, including yourself, which builds a negative bias into your observations, identifications and questioning. Interviewed perspectives are therefore due the same respect you expect to receive from others.

Additionally, if I assume you are a symbol, as I may if you appear in one of my dreams, I am focusing on your meaning for me and on your instrumental value in my life. Your being is derived from and dependent upon the meanings that I project upon it. This constitutes a subtle discount of your value because I am making your existence secondary to my interpretations, meanings and values. However, when I suspend my reality claims for myself and for you and simply experience who and what you are, I thereby acknowledge your integrity as a separate being. While interviewed elements obviously do not possess the same reality that you do (for instance, they don't possess physical bodies), *to approach them as if they do possess the same reality* is both important and valuable. Such an approach is fundamental to phenomenalistic orientations, and it is foundational to IDL.

A way to understand your patterns of personal preference

If meeting a problem externally is suffering, then resolving that same problem internally, before it is externalized, is grace at work. Intention is a mysterious, primal, and magical force that shines through natural, human, and transpersonal dimensions of being. Whether viewed as predetermined or free, everywhere you look, from the indeterminacy of Heisenberg's electrons to the deepest meditation of Gautama Buddha, you will find patterns of prepersonal, personal, and transpersonal preference, as manifestations of intention. Even among atoms we find preferences. For example, oxygen atoms "prefer" ten electrons but only have eight, and hydrogen atoms "prefer" two electrons but only have one. Atoms "satisfy their yearnings" by sharing electrons.[8] This is because intention is an innate aspect of consciousness, perception and experience and cannot be escaped, either intrasocially or as a projection onto society.

Intention expresses itself in form as preference. This means that while pure intention transcends preference, in the world of perspectives, ideas, and feelings, it has gradations. Preferences structure reality and determine experience. Your awareness of your available preferences determines your choices in life.[9] Unresolved conflicting preferences, whether known or unknown to you, block your development and are experienced as suffering. Awareness of your preferences is freedom; ignorance of those preferences that condition your experience and are obstructions to your development is suffering.[10] Awareness of your preferences is a prerequisite to their eventual transcendence through identification with a compassionate knowingness that is one with all conditioning preferences.

Your preferences change based on your level of development, line of development, holon quadrant, state, and the particular phase of your developmental dialectic that you are transitioning.[11] For example, your decision to learn *Dream Sociometry* is a preference. In its internal individual aspect, it is an intent. Internally and collectively, it is a particular value that you like, like a lot, love, dislike, dislike a lot, hate, or feel neutral about. You may feel some combination of these degrees of preference. In addition, you give meanings to your preferences, and these meanings are also aspects of the internal collective quadrant of your human holon. An example of a meaning is to see learning Dream Sociometry as a way to broaden your understanding of IDL, speed your own development, and hopefully serve others more effectively. The external individual aspect of your preference is manifested by your behavior, what you are doing now: reading about Dream Sociometry. The external collective aspect of this preference involves the impact that your decision to learn Dream Sociometry will have on those who come into contact with you.

Just as you have preferences, so do your interviewed emerging potentials. Does your lack of awareness of their preferences mean that they do not have an impact on your life? Does it mean that their preferences are less relevant or important than your own? On the contrary, *the preferences of your interviewed emerging potentials have a profound and ongoing impact on every aspect of your life, whether you are aware of them or not.* This is partially because the preferences held by some invested perspectives naturally conflict with other invested perspectives. Notice that in order to be invested, a perspective does not have to be "yours." Instead, it can be a *potential* that is emerging into your awareness for the first time. Perhaps it is the combination of new relationships and associations that you have never before made.

When disruptive conflicts are not recognized, understood, neutralized, or integrated into a higher-order synthesis, they may create confusion and disease. They can block both your personal and transpersonal development. If you are unable to resolve destructive conflicts, in time, they may be projected externally onto your body and your life experiences, as well as onto your relationships with others. This is because conflicts that are significant don't go away; they can become louder and more intrusive. Dream characters may model reactivity and fear, creating anxiety as you sleep.

Nightmares can be viewed as expressions of internal conflict personified as warring internal preferences. When you have nightmares your body is experiencing the Alarm Stage of what Hans Selye described as the General Adaptation Syndrome. Adrenaline and powerful neurotransmitters evoke a physiological response within your sympathetic nervous system that eats at the sleeping systems of your body like battery acid. These highly toxic hormones and enzymes cannot be discharged through either fight or flight during dream sleep because your voluntary muscles are naturally paralyzed, so you don't act out your dreams while sleeping and hurt yourself. Your health is undone as the toxic byproducts of stressful dreams cannot be eliminated through fight or flight; you awaken on edge, yet you may have no recollection of the dream, a victim of your unknown distal selves.[12]

If you ignore your nightmares, your wake-up calls may get louder. One way of doing so is by *externalizing* – moving from the land of nightmares to the realm of waking nightmare, manifesting commonly as drama and pathologically as post-traumatic stress disorder. The problematic people and events you attract to yourself can therefore often be usefully considered as externalizations of your unresolved internal conflicts.[13] When you ignore your interior preferences, they may get louder by eventually manifesting as waking, somnambulistic dreams. What is ignored within may eventually be projected without in a form that cannot be ignored.

External conflicts are both more difficult to avoid and generally more painful to resolve than internal ones, yet because they are inherently subjective we typically lack the objectivity to first recognize them and then intervene in effective ways. Much pain between individuals, within businesses, and among nations can be avoided when conflicts are addressed at their roots – within the individuals involved. In health care, this is one form of "upstream prevention." If you can understand and address etiology you save time, money, and misery in downstream crisis intervention. In IDL, this is done when you listen to and resolve conflicting internal preferences.

When viewed from a Dream Sociometric perspective, your intrasocial groups metaphorically depict not only psychological patterns at work within you but transpersonal intent as well. As you practice Dream Sociometry, these basic patterns become clear and their implications for your future evident. Once this knowledge becomes available, it becomes easier for you to stop victimizing yourself. Once you learn to identify with perspectives that personify healthy preferences, you experience yourself making better choices in what you feel, think, and do. This is a fundamental, foundational type of growth that is generalized rather than limited to.one area of your life. The impact is likely to be substantial, rather than a passing insight or experience. Fundamental transformation is normally experienced as increased self-awareness, reduced suffering, increased life satisfaction, or improved problem-solving ability. As you continue to consult with your interviewed emerging potentials, the reduction in the amount, type, and intensity of conflict among them will validate a growing sense that the changes you are experiencing are indeed genuine and profound.

Dream Sociometry is more than a process of gaining knowledge of those preferences that condition your existence and impact on your health and performance today. You will come in contact with perspectives whose world view transcends all preferences. One such emerging potential is Dream Consciousness, that hypothesized perspective that creates your dreams. IDL does not care whether Dream Consciousness is "real" or not, but focuses on the function of taking its perspective. By experiencing your dreams and life dramas from its world view, you learn how to witness multiple invested preferences with unusual objectivity, which creates a liberating sense of detachment from your life drama. "The Great Way is not difficult for those who have no preferences."[14]

Description of the method

The Dream Sociometric *method* is a series of steps or injunctions:

- Think of three fundamental life issues that you are presently concerned about. Write them down.
- Write your dream or life experience in 1st-person present tense. This can be a composite life experience: for instance, an imaginary summation of many instances of abandonment or stage fright.
- Write your associations to the dream or life experience, if any. This is where you take your best stab at what you think the dream or life experience "means," that is, what role it has played in your life script to create the person you are today. If it was a dream, perhaps you are sure it is due to that movie you saw last night. Perhaps you are certain it is meaningless. In any case, note your associations.
- Create a data collection grid called the *Dream Sociomatrix*. List *chosen* characters, actions, and feelings, together called "elements," chronologically across the top of the Dream Sociomatrix. List *choosing* characters down the left-hand margin. In choosing interviewed characters, express preferences regarding chosen interviewed characters, actions, and feelings.
- Imagine yourself back in the dream or life experience, taking the role of each chosen character in succession.

- As each character, express as written numerical values your preferences regarding how you feel about yourself in the dream (called "Dream Self"), your companions, and what is going on in the dream.

- Seven orders of preference, *love, like a lot, like, neutrality, dislike, dislike a lot,* and *hate* are used, with the corresponding numerical values of 3, 2, 1, 0, -1, -2, and -3. Each stated preference is written in the grid as its corresponding numerical value. A final preference, *transcendence of preferences,* is sometimes marked with a dot "•" but has no numerical value and is not plotted in the Dream Sociogram.

- Elaborations, which are interviewed character statements that explain their preferences, are noted in the *Dream Sociomatrix Commentary.*

- Particularly significant statements may be underlined for restatement later as "I" statements.

- The dreamer has an opportunity to express what, if anything, has surprised him in what he has heard his interviewed characters say.

- Each interviewed character is then asked how it would change the dream (or waking life situation) if it could change it in any way it wanted – as long as all other interviewed characters have no objection to any proposed change. The comments of each interviewed character are written in the *Dreamage Commentary.*

- From this information, a reorganized dream may be created, known as a "*Dreamage.*" This is possible only if all interviewed characters agree on the changes suggested by interviewed characters.

- Each interviewed character is asked what aspect of the dreamer it most closely personifies, why it is in the dream, and why this particular intrasocial group came together. This information is written in the *Dream Summary Commentary.*

- Each interviewed character is asked how it would change the dreamer's waking life if that interviewed character were living the dreamer's day-to-day existence. Responses are written in the *Waking Commentary.*

- Each interviewed character is then asked to consider how it would handle each of your three life issues.

- In the *Identification Commentary,* your interviewed characters are given the opportunity to indicate in what specific waking situations it would be most helpful for you to imagine that you are them.

- An *Action Plan* based on those recommendations that are acceptable to waking identity is created. It is intended to act as a guide to daily application of life changes suggested and supported by interviewed perspectives.

- An additional, optional step creates a picture of the intrasocial patterns of preference manifesting themselves in a particular dream. This map of consciousness is called a *Dream Sociogram.* The creation and interpretation of Dream Sociograms is explained in Dillard, J. *Understanding the Dream Sociogram.*

- An explanatory commentary on the Dream Sociogram may be added, called the *Dream Group Dynamics Commentary*.
- The interviewed characters may also be asked what you can do differently to avoid repeating previous mistakes in your life and for direction in fulfilling the priorities of your life compass. This step is called creating the *Transpersonal Growth Commentary*.
- You may rephrase core remarks of the interviewed characters in the commentaries in first person, present tense in a section called, "What I am saying to myself is . . ."
- The fundamental issues expressed by the intrasocial group are summarized.
- The dreamer consults characters appearing in subsequent dreams or waking life derived sociomatrices for their feedback regarding the dreamer's understanding and application of their daily Action Plan.
- The usefulness of these efforts is monitored and evaluated by feedback from successive interviewed perspectives, waking identity and external support systems, particularly IDL peers, called the waking IDL Sangha.

Rationale

Each of the above steps has its own rationale.

- Writing the dream in 1st-person present tense helps you to experience the dream as if it is happening to you now. This assists in identifying with the experience.
- Writing your associations serves as a pre-test so that you can objectively evaluate any changes to your understanding of your dream.
- To get the most out of your work, you need to experience its relevance and usefulness in relationship to current concerns in your life. This is why three life issues are identified at the beginning of the process.
- The Dream Sociomatrix is a grid used to collect character preferences. It provides a method of objectifying largely unrecognized preferences that precipitate out as elements and their relationships in your dreams and waking life.
- Becoming different elements allows you to disidentify with your typical waking perspective, in which you tend to be stuck, and to broaden your view of your life through experiencing and witnessing more objective perspectives that are experienced as authentic and viable.
- In addition to putting you in touch with a wide variety of otherwise easily overlooked perspectives that are invested in your dream or life drama, assigning a degree of preference to your experiences as an interviewed element also stimulates thoughts and feelings that explain these preferences.
- Predicting patterns of preference that will be expressed by the various interviewed element provides an optional pre-test to gauge your waking

ability to accurately assess inner perspectives. These predictions can be compared with the actual preferences that reveal themselves in the Dream Sociomatrix. These are: "most accepting, character," most rejecting character," "most preferred character/action/feeling," and "most rejected character-action-feeling."

- When you write elaborations of element preferences in the *Dream Sociomatrix Commentary*, you give voice to valuable but largely ignored perspectives. This information can be both revelatory and useful.

- Underlining particularly important statements makes sure that they are repeated later as "I" statements, in which you own, or take responsibility for, what you have said to yourself in the voice of this or that interviewed perspective.

- Commenting on what is surprising about the above elaborations creates a historical record of what is being heard and what is being learned that is new and different. These often include significant shifts in awareness and perspective.

- Asking the various interviewed elements how they would change the dream provides an opportunity to view an idealized alteration of intrasocial dynamics from the perspective of other emerging potentials. The resulting rewritten dream is a visual metaphor that may have implications that are very different from those of the original dream or your own idealized sense of how you would change a dream or a life drama. For example, in a nightmare of being chased by a monster, your preferred change might be that the monster disappears, but other interviewed elements might want to change the dream so that you listen to what the monster says and does. These are two different proposed outcomes and each has vastly different implications for your development. Because you are receiving recommendations from many more emerging potentials that you typically do in an IDL interview, you are more likely to arrive at rewritten dreams that depict how different interest groups would like to see themselves evolve.

- Dreamages are metaphors of internal integration that have the combined weight of all your interviewed elements behind them. The purpose of the dreamage is to reprogram your awareness using an innate and powerful experience of integration that inherently speaks deeply to you. Because many perspectives are consulted, any agreed-upon dreamage is much more likely to reflect a broad consensus of internal support. Such an image of internally desirable integration has powerful therapeutic implications and uses.

- Asking your interviewed elements what aspects of yourself they most closely personify is a way to have them provide their own interpretation for who and what they are in your life. While not replacing other interpretive resources, such interpretations clearly claim a priority and an authority inaccessible to less direct interpretive methods, such as symbol interpretation books and experts. Because you are enquiring regarding a cross-section of the elements that appear in the dream or life drama, you have a clearer sense of how your consciousness uses form to express multiple authentic perspectives on your life.

- Just as your interviewed elements have definite ideas about how they would change your dream or life drama, they usually have specific suggestions about how they would change your life if they were running it instead of you. Such recommendations provide novel and creative approaches to waking life change. Because you are interviewing many more emerging potentials than you typically do in the IDL single-element interviewing protocol processes, you will generally receive many more recommendations for improving your life.
- Concrete suggestions provided by your interviewed elements about how they would handle your three life issues provide practical guidance and direction regarding concerns that matter to you from sources that know you intimately.
- Waking identification with your interviewed elements in specific life situations allows you to put IDL to the test. What changes occur in your life? Do related problem situations become better or worse? Because the element interviewing process is more in depth than it is in single-element interviewing, you have identified with more perspectives for a longer period of time. This means that your waking identifications are likely to be deeper and more natural.
- Your Action Plan culls all of the recommendations made by various interviewed elements and places them in one section where they can be reviewed and adopted or discarded, as desired.
- The Dream Sociogram depicts the interviewed element preferences tabulated in the Dream Sociomatrix in such a way that the patterns of preference of the entire group are exhibited. This provides a way of forming conclusions about your level, lines, quadrants, states and stage of self-development as well as that of your various interviewed elements. This information is largely inaccessible through the single-element interviewing protocol.
- The purpose of the rephrasing of earlier underlined elaborations as "I" statements is to help you fully own the perspectives that have been expressed by interviewed elements. Practice in reading over "I" statements is an enormous aid to the thoughtful and cogent reading back of element statements to students as "I" statements.
- Summarization of interviewed element issues provides a sort of "post-test" by which you can compare your initial "pre-test" associations with what you have learned from completing the Dream Sociomatrix.
- The interpretive elaborations of IDL teachers, Practitioners, and students and the ongoing support of subsequent interviewed elements is important in creating a congruency of inner and outer experience so that your growth becomes richer and deeper.

Summary

- Dream Sociometry is a foundational, generally self-directed and thorough approach to IDL interviewing. It provides a powerful personal research tool for the healing, balancing, and expansion of consciousness.
- Dream Sociometry uses element identification as a way to gain objectivity and to cultivate the witness.
- It interviews multiple perspectives from the same dream or life situation in order to access perspectives that can help you align your life with the agenda of your life compass.
- Dream Sociometry provides in-depth knowledge of many of the processes used more superficially in IDL single-element interviewing protocols.

Notes

1 These can be found at IntegralDeepListening.Com, "Questionnaires."
2 Conflicts only exist from prepersonal and personal perspectives, not from transpersonal perspectives. Conflict and its resolution is one perceptual stance used by IDL as assumptions associated with normal prepersonal and personal level perception. From transpersonal perspectives, conflicts are transcended and integrated into larger wholes. Transpersonal perspectives are not, however, "better" than prepersonal or personal perspectives just because they transcend and include them. Nor does this mean that conflict does not "really" exist, just as it is false to say that perspectives that transcend conflict are delusions. When a child is learning to walk, trigonometry is of no help whatsoever. Similarly, in the everyday reality of prepersonal and personal level existence, conflict is real enough, and to minimize it by affirming that "all is in divine order" or that conflict is part of "dharmic destiny," karma, or some divine plan, is both reductionistic and cruel. How the experience o-f conflict changes with developmental perspective is an illustration of how IDL emphasizes multi-perspectivalism. There are life situations where you need to recognize and respond to conflict if you want to grow or even stay alive, for example, the conflict between staying alert or falling asleep when driving long distances at night. Similarly, there are life situations when you want and need to affirm and experience transcending, integral perspectives. Most of life involves the former, but the latter creates and maintains a necessary context for moment-to-moment enlightenment.
3 Whether or not IDL can accurately be called a "yoga" when development takes students past mid-transpersonal or subtle levels of evolution is a matter of speculation. In the causal realms and beyond, there is no self to be united with anything, and the union of self and the divine or whole is the classical definition of yoga. The self as an ontological being or substance is in fact transcended at causal and non-dual, as are all subject-object dualisms. However, IDL remains a yoga in the sense that it is a transpersonal integral life practice or injunctive methodology, that continues to provide support as long as humans continue to evolve.
4 While "object permanence," a term popularized by cognitive psychologist Piaget, who specialized in childhood development, indicates the ability to understand that people and things remain when one closes their eyes or is no longer looking at them, subject permanence is, on the one hand, the awareness that no matter where your body is or what feelings you experience or thoughts you think, there is a consistent sense of beingness, presence, and "I amness." On the other hand, subject permanence is the ability to objectify that self, or "witness the witness" as an ongoing, background awareness.

5 Students come to understand through their study of IDL that the assumptions that they make about the relative reality of both waking and dreaming are subjective, arbitrary, and, while functionally necessary to do work in the world, have no fundamental reality or *bhava*, "own being," to use the Buddhist term. This is learned through applying IDL to waking events in the same way that it is applied to dream experience and finding that the results are phenomenologically the same. While you and I necessarily do so, life itself simply does not distinguish between waking and dreaming experience in any substantial way. The consequence of this understanding is that the "dream" that is referred to in "dream yoga," is discovered to be *experience itself* and the world of form, whether encountered while awake, dreaming, meditating, or any other realm of being.

6 The negative scores are written as "/1," "/2," or "/3," rather than as "−1," "−2," or "−3" for ease of reading in the Dream Sociomatrix.

7 Concepts from Wilber's *Integral Psychology* (Shambala, Boston, 2000), as well as many of his other works, are used throughout texts on IDL, with the most thorough discussion of them to be found in *Transformational Dreamwork*.

8 Packard, Edward, *Imagining the Universe,* Berkeley Pub., NY., 1994, p. 106. Such anthropomorphizing is a form of elevationism. As long as this is remembered and such analogies are taken metaphorically, they can be helpful.

9 While "choice" is an emotionally neutral underlying component of preference, it is quite difficult and unusual to find choices that are not either influenced by or manifestations of, emotion. It is our identification with our emotions, generally out of our awareness, as our subtle preferences, that are a major source of both confusion and suffering. Because Dream Sociometry is invested in the reduction of suffering as a pre-requisite to the advancement of most forms of clarity, it emphasizes preference in its sociometric structure. However, other parts of IDL, particularly script analysis and the recognition and elimination of cognitive distortions emphasize choice.

10 All conflict is not suffering. On a cellular and systemic basis, homeostasis is maintained by conflicting preferences that lie mostly out of our awareness. These conflicts are *resolved* in the sense that they do not create suffering because they interact in a higher order synthesis, even if they do create adaptational challenges necessary for growth and development. We normally habituate to various routines, like walking and driving, which play themselves out largely as automatic scripts while masquerading as conscious awareness. Moving from one habitual routine to the next, waking identity is largely somnambulistic and without the experience of either conflict or suffering.

11 These are concepts from Wilber's Integral AQAL and are amplified in Dillard, J. (2002). *Transformational Dreamwork*. Berlin: Integral Deep Listening Press.

12 "Distal" selves are the roles you play and that you witness with your "proximal self."

13 This does not mean that the people and events that you experience that are conflictual or traumatic *are* externalizations of internal conflict, but only that it is useful to view them as such. IDL does not claim to know what external things *really* are. It does not disclose the *ding an sich*, or "thing in itself," to use Kant's phrase, yet it does not claim that things are fundamentally illusory, even though they are dreamlike. This is because a dream is real enough when you are dreaming it; a lucid dream is real enough when you are acting within it knowing you are dreaming; life is real enough when you are stuck in circumstances that are beyond your control.

14 The Third Patriarch of Zen.

Bibliography

Dillard, J. (2002). *Transformational dreamwork*. Berlin: Integral Deep Listening Press.

Wilber, K. (2000). *Integral psychology*. Boston: Shambala.

Chapter 2

Benefits of Dream Sociometry

Dream Sociometry is a transpersonal methodology because it is not centered on any definition of self whatsoever. It is not centered on ego, an altruistic, compassionate self, on soul, Self, or *Atman*. It is not centered on a definition of self as one with all. It is not psychologically geocentric but rather *polycentric*, or *multi-perspectival*. Every point and every perspective interviewed or capable of being interviewed is, without exception, the center of experience. This does not fit nicely into any of the four traditional definitions of the transpersonal, oneness with nature, deity, formlessness, or the non-dual because these all deal with degrees of selflessness and varieties of oneness. Dream Sociometry and IDL both assumes and generates selflessness and varieties of oneness equally within prepersonal, personal, and transpersonal contexts.

As such, it is a methodology, an empirical method, a yoga, an injunctive path, and an integral life practice. What makes it a *transpersonal* methodology is that it is not directed by the goals of self, as are most empirical methods, yogas, injunctive paths, or integral life practices. Instead, it is directed by a combination of common sense, the advice of respected others, and intrasocial sources of objectivity, as represented by the recommendations of interviewed emerging potentials. This can be differentiated by the usual appeals to direction by God, dharma, intuition, conscience, life guides, and scripture by an operationally defined description: IDL defines your life compass as consensus recommendations for life change from a variety of interviewed emerging potentials. Therefore, "life compass" for IDL is a process, not a thing.

Provides an unrivaled depth of understanding about any and every dream

Almost all approaches to understanding dreams come either from the perspective of the dreamer or outside interpreters, whether in intrasocial groups, therapy, Scripture, and symbology dictionaries. These are all exterior and therefore projective. Their interpretations are projections of their experience and point of view. They may think they know you better than you know yourself and believe that they are fully capable of disclosing your blind spots. Perhaps they are! However, the basic problem is that others don't know you and *can't* know you as well as any of the perspectives interviewed by IDL, because *they aren't you*. They also lack the unique objectivity that these perspectives provide

Eliminates nightmares

While IDL single character interviewing also eliminates nightmares, Dream Sociometry does so even more quickly and completely. This is because of the depth and thoroughness with which the etiology of the disturbance is not only understood, but the multiple recommendations for attitudinal and behavioral change that reduce nightmare-inducing factors. The main reason why IDL is so effective at eliminating nightmares is because it reframes them in ways that are not only no longer threatening, but generally seen as positive, supportive and therapeutic. Most but not all of the time, this simple reframing is so effective that it is all that is required, even with long-term, repetitive nightmares.

Generates powerful and profound new recognitions of the relationship between dreaming and waking experience

When you create sociomatrices and sociograms of waking nightmares or childhood wounds that have been buried or never resolved, you quickly discover that waking life events are structured like dreams and have similar characteristics, when viewed from the perspectives of interviewed characters. This teaches you to look at your own personal traumas and nightmares as dreams while giving you insight into the specific mechanisms that perpetuate their hold over your life.

Brings new depth of understanding to both dreams and waking dreams

This depth is largely due to an increase in self-acceptance, based on a new and clearer recognition that the majority of invested perspectives that you interview are much more accepting of yourself and your circumstances than you are. However, those which are in fact *less* accepting generally have good and equally clear reasons why they are not accepting. Therefore, instead of treating dreams and waking life as symbolic events, to be interpreted, or as conflicts to be resolved, IDL interviewing of multiple perspectives in Dream Sociometry teaches you to view both objectively, from perspectives that are relatively free of your life scripting, addictions, drama, and cognitive distortions.

Discloses normally unrecognized conflict

We normally assume one role and then another consecutively in our daily lives. Separation in time and context make us oblivious to contradictory and conflicting expectations, assumptions, preferences, and behaviors among our different roles. For instance, our work may require us to be predatory, ruthless, manipulative, or dishonest, although we rarely recognize this to be the case, in order to protect our self-image. However, at home and in our community the expectation is that we are loving partners and parents as well as responsible citizens. Many, many people routinely live their lives with a basic contradiction in values without ever realizing it, such is the magic of the separation of roles based on time and context. Because the creation of a Dream Sociomatrix brings roles normally separated by time and context into a shared context in the here and now, any conflict among our roles becomes obvious. This is an extremely valuable recognition if our intent is to align our priorities with those of our inner compass and reduce misery, suffering, and pain. However, most of the time, most of us are more or less comfortable with our circumstances. There may be an issue here or there we want to change, but we have spent considerable time and effort building our roles and the lifestyle they support. Therefore, it is not to be assumed that uncovering and resolving underlying core conflicts is something that any of us will do without encountering significant resistance.

Discloses the transpersonal

Dream Sociometry provides both temporary state access to all four transpersonal states as well as an instructional methodology, as a variety of IDL, itself a form of dream yoga, that develops fundamental components of transpersonal experience.[1] These include the decentralization of self through multiperspectivalism; non-personalization through identification with multiple perspectives; witnessing through the cultivation of objectivity as these various perspectives, empathy through observing life and dream dramas from the perspectives of others; wisdom; and transcendence of dualities, acceptance, compassion, inner peace, and confidence. It teaches and strongly recommends meditation as a part of its integral life practice.

Recognizes role conflicts by interviewing multiple invested perspectives

When you interview perspectives that personify your misery, whether physical or mental/emotional, and then interview perspectives that personify the secondary gains that you receive by maintaining your misery, your predicament generally becomes clear. Parts of you want to get well, while other parts want to stay sick! Fortunately, almost every interview will also disclose perspectives that are relatively clear of both misery and secondary gain and that therefore provide objectivity that is vital for finding your way forward.

Addresses disclosed conflicts in a self-directed, therapeutic way

When you interview a number of perspectives at the same time the differences in their world views, as well as the solutions they provide, are intrasocial; they are not provided by other people. Therefore, you are challenged with the responsibility of having to sort through issues that are clearly self-generated. This teaches both personal responsibility and personal empowerment. The Dream Sociogram provides a perspective on conflict that is inherently therapeutic because it is objective and therefore relatively devoid of drama.

Increases self-acceptance by encountering perspectives that are much less self-critical than you are

While you will encounter self-critical perspectives when you do Dream Sociometry, you will generally encounter many more perspectives that are less critical of you than you are. As a result of identifying with such perspectives and understanding their reasons for their acceptance, you will have a tendency over time and with the creation of a number of Dream Sociograms, to increase your acceptance of yourself. This is critically important, because self-acceptance is fundamental for mental health.

Supports transpersonal development by teaching multi-perspectivalism

Multi-perspectivalism creates a polycentric rather than a geocentric identity. Polycentric identities are inherently transpersonal because they are no longer about defining reality in relationship to a fixed sense of identity. There is no longer one, unitary self that is "real"; instead, there are a multiplicity of authentic and legitimate perspectives, all of which reveal truth and reality. The result is the inevitable thinning and broadening of the self, which is the fundamental characteristic of the transpersonal.

Supports transpersonal development by cultivating empathy

Empathy is defined as the ability to look at the world from the perspectives of others. IDL character identification is immersion training in empathy and creating Dream Sociomatrices brings that training to a graduate level by requiring the ability to smoothly shift from one identity to another at depth, time after time throughout the creation of the various commentaries. The more you increase your ability to empathize with disgusting, bizarre, stupid, or pointless perspectives, the more your identity becomes transpersonal. This is because you no longer identify with particular characteristics that define who and what you are, such as purity, rationality, intelligence, or purpose.

Increases confidence in interviewing through increasing your depth of knowledge

Learning to create Dream Sociomatrices and Sociograms brings your interviewing ability to a completely different level of understanding and competency. Consequently, regular IDL single interviews of dream characters and the personifications of life issues will become both easier and more understandable, with the result being that your confidence in your ability to not only interview, but to help students of IDL learn and grow with IDL, will increase.

Provides a professional depth of expertise behind and supporting your practice

Anyone can find copies of IDL interviewing protocols on line or elsewhere and begin using them with themselves and others. In fact, we encourage others to do so, with or without attribution. However, cultivating a professional depth to practice requires experience with creating Dream Sociomatrices and Sociograms. The difference in competency between those who have done so and those who have not is apparent.

Creating dreamages demonstrates how internal consensus supports both integration and powerful decision making

Dreamages cannot be forced on any group of choosers. However, when they themselves agree to the description of a dream, the sense of integration standing behind that particular visual metaphor is palpable. It is one thing to arrive at a decision yourself; it is quite another thing to arrive at decisions with the support of multiple authentic and relatively autonomous perspectives. Such decisions feel different and carry stronger intention and conviction forward in their implementation.

Differences from single-character interviewing

Collects much more information of a very high quality

Dream Sociometry normally interviews four or five characters and Dream Consciousness. This provides a wealth of data from the stating of preferences and the explanations for them that are provided. The questions of each successive commentary are answered by all characters and the relationships between all of them are displayed on the Dream Sociogram. The result is a smorgasbord of rich and multi-layered understanding not only about how and why you are stuck but what you need to do to get unstuck. Compare the results to other narrative tools for self-discovery that you are familiar with, such as Meyers-Briggs, *I Ching*, astrology charts, and enneagrams, and draw your own conclusions.

Interviews several emerging potentials at a time (multi-perspectival)

We have seen how the interviewing of multiple perspectives speeds up the deconstruction of the unitary, psychologically geocentric, self. Doing so also provides multiple inputs for problem-solving from perspectives that are invested and knowledgeable, yet are not stuck in the scripting, drama, and cognitive distortions that we are.

Encouragement of autonomy

You only properly identify with a particular interviewed character when you honestly speak from its perspective. This same principle is also essential to the effectiveness of Moreno's sociometry and psychodrama.[2] When you do so, you will find that interviewed characters often exercise great autonomy, presenting specific opinions widely divergent from your waking viewpoint. Consequently, merging with interviewed characters can be an eye-opening and humbling experience. In one commentary, *An Eggcellent Chicken Operation*, I am scolded by several interviewed characters for spending too much time doing dreamwork! What is paradoxical about this is that if I hadn't been creating Dream Sociomatrices, I never would have heard this complaint!

Such interviewing discloses the relative independence of emerging potentials without assuming that they possess completely separate existence. As holons, they are both self and other, interior and exterior. Becoming successive interviewed characters as you create a Dream Sociomatrix increases your contact with reality by broadening your interpretive contexts; it represents a movement *away* from dissociation. Its purpose is to emphasize and expand the interdependent nature of your entire being. You share awareness and power with multiple legitimate alternative perspectives. As you identify with other interior and subjective points of view that are nevertheless exterior and objective to your sense of self, you accept and integrate them into an expanded experience of who you are. Consequently, healing, balancing, and transformation occur as you fill out the Dream Sociomatrix and elicit interviewed character elaborations.

Dream Self is interviewed

Dream Sociometry interviews your perspective in a dream or in a waking life situation, called "Dream Self," as a baseline of preference against which the perspectives of other interviewed characters can be compared. It also consults Dream Self regarding every commentary question in order to integrate the various perspectives provided into the framework of your current self-sense. These procedures provide important and valuable support for growth that are not available in single-character interviewing.

Used when growth requires the appreciation of multiple perspectives

While childhood is largely about the building of a unitary self-sense and adulthood is about the using of that self to provide meaningful service in the world, there is no age that is too early or cannot benefit from exposure to multiple perspectives. We already recognize this in the benefits to babies who are exposed to multiple parental figures and to animals. Even young children can eliminate nightmares by taking on the perspectives of monsters, dream threats, and attackers. Input from multiple perspectives stabilizes and integrates the thesis stage of development while making the resolution of conflicts raised in the antithesis stage smoother and easier. Both of these together make synthesis, or graduation to a permanent higher level of development, more likely.

Increases detachment from preferences

Our preferences largely anchor us to a mid-prepersonal level of development. This is because they define happiness and personal fulfillment in terms of getting what we want and avoiding what we don't want while avoiding getting what we don't want and not getting what we want. This approach to life means we doom ourselves to unhappiness when we get what we don't want and separate ourselves from what we do want. Eliciting multiple preferences from multiple perspectives in the Dream Sociogram tends to distance us first from our own preferences and then from preferences in general. This means that preferences still exist and we continue to have likes and dislikes, but their ability to define who we are and what creates happiness and misery diminishes. This translates into a freedom from drama and increased emotional objectivity. We continue to have strong feelings, but they no longer define us.

Does not ask for scores using the six core qualities

In the single-character interviewing protocols, interviewed perspectives are asked to score themselves, zero to ten, in confidence, empathy, wisdom, acceptance, inner peace, and witnessing. These qualities provide multiple dimensions by which to evaluate where the perspectives score themselves in these qualities and why. It also allows us to experience what it would be like to score in a similar way. In Dream Sociometry, so much other work is being done on identifying and objectifying preferences and conflict that scoring in the six core qualities is unnecessary. However, there is no reason why it cannot be done; you are free to experiment with doing so if you desire.

Interviews dream consciousness, providing a relatively objective and contextual perspective on life drama

Dream Consciousness is the name IDL gives to the perspective of the context or set which includes the subset of all interviewed perspectives, including Dream Self. As such, it adds another level of witnessing and objectivity to the process. The first level comes with the writing of the narrative; the second is in the expression of any associations one has to it; the third is in the objectifying of Dream Self's preferences in the Sociomatrix; the fourth is in the elaborations of those preferences; the fifth is in the objectifying of the preferences of other interviewed perspectives; the sixth is in the elaborations that explain their preferences; the seventh is in the answers to the various commentaries; the eighth is in the preferences provided by Dream Consciousness; and the ninth is in its elaborations that explain its preferences and its remarks in the various commentaries. The tenth is the objectivity provided by the various elements, including Dream Consciousness, in the Dream Sociomatrix. The eleventh is the objectivity of your perspective as observer of all interviewed perspectives, including Dream Consciousness, as they are positioned in the Dream Sociogram.

Creates dreamages

Dreamages are not possible in single-character interviews because they are consensus creations of multiple interviewed perspectives.

Creates dream sociograms

Dream Sociograms provide a visual representation of the relationships created by the patterns of preference expressed by the various interviewed characters in the Dream Sociomatrix. These patterns are normally invisible because Dream Self is identified with *its* preferences and is blind not only to those of others but to the relationships created among various preferences. This blindness can be verified by attempting to predict most and least preferring choosers and chosen elements or to attempt to create an accurate Dream Sociogram before any characters are interviewed.

Discloses intrasocial dynamics

Whether you are dealing with patterns of preferences among dream characters or those what are invested in a life issue, patterns are created that disclose unsuspected relationships among perspectives that are not always right or thoughtful but almost always enlightening.

Discloses developmental dynamics

Development occurs through a dialectic of thesis, antithesis, and synthesis. All are necessary, which means that conflict is as important and beneficial as its absence. Consequently, the purpose of IDL is not to resolve or eliminate conflict, but to listen to it as a wake-up call. Normally, this act of respect eliminates conflict, but not always. For example, IDL does not magically make cancer or chronic disease go away just by respectfully listening to the various perspectives invested in the disease. However, such deep and respectful listening to multiple invested perspectives will allow you to place your pain and suffering into an authentic nurturing and supportive context which provides and supports a profound definition of healing, one that can include and transcend death.

Provides many more recommendations for your integral life practice

Interviewing five or six characters, all of which are generally opinionated, will produce an abundance of recommendations. You have to first list them so that you can decide which ones you want to act on. You then need to figure out how to operationalize them, to define them in such a way that change can be measured. This provides you with a means of knowing whether your application of recommendations is helpful or not, both for your own development and to develop your trust and confidence in IDL.

Learning to withdraw waking projections

It is natural for you to project your meanings onto your intrasocial groups, since you routinely project your meanings onto your waking experiences and relationships. For example, if you have trouble trusting yourself, it follows that you may find many people's motives and actions questionable. If you are unreliable, is it surprising that you find that you can't rely on others? If you are critical of others, is it a surprise to find that you are also self-critical? Similarly, whether you think that dreams are literal, visionary and truthful, your dreams will tend to validate your assumptions, just as they will if you assume that they are symbolic, regressive, and illusory. If you look for particular dream symbols or archetypes, is it so amazing that you find them? Consequently, your interpretations of all experience, particularly your dreams, inevitably reflect your biases. As a consequence, you gain precious little new information about the dream itself from your interpretations. Similarly, the interpretations of others not only reflect their biases and projections, but collective cultural assumptions and world views of which they are largely unaware. One has to be completely outside the cultural context, as we are when we view, say, ancient Egyptian or Tibetan Buddhist dream interpretation, to appreciate just how projective of waking assumptions dream interpretation is.

It is much more important but far less common to allow life – whether encountered awake or in a dream – to express *itself* to you. The Dream Socio-matrix is designed to allow this fascinating process to occur. As a phenomenalis-tic methodology, identifying with interviewed characters while creating Dream Sociomatrices encourages you to set your waking biases and interpretations aside for the moment. When you do, you observe different points of view in the form of interviewed character preferences regarding issues that are significant in your life. In *The Hanging Corpse*, one of a series of over 50 Dream Sociomatrices and Commentaries that the author drew from in creating this text, Dream Self is confronted by his own guilt in the metaphorical form of knowledge that he killed part of himself and stuffed it deep down inside. In waking life, he was running away from this awareness. It took a nightmarish dream to wake him up.

Character identification during the creation of the Dream Sociomatrix invites multiple perspectives to take responsibility for being in the dream, for their stake in its action and outcome. In expressing its preferences, each inter-viewed character is projecting *its* biases and interpretations onto the dream and, therefore, onto your life.

Summary

* The above list of benefits of Dream Sociometry are not meant to be accepted by you out of hand. Rather, they are to be tested and evaluated in the laboratory of your own life and integral life practice.
* It is only by creating both Dream Sociomatrices and doing single dream and life issue interviews that you can evaluate the comparisons mentioned above and decide which make sense to you.

Notes

1 What makes something transpersonal? First, it must include the prepersonal and the per-sonal. These can be defined in many ways, but most basically, they are developmental stages that reflect growth in at least four core lines: cognition, self-awareness, morality, and empathy. These develop within four quadrants of the human holon, society, culture, behavior, and consciousness. A picture of these relationships is included below. The prep-ersonal is associated with early stages of social collectives (familial, tribal) and organization (foraging, horticultural, agrarian), cultural (archaic, magic, and belief), behavioral (atomic, molecular and physiological structures and processes), and consciousness (prehension, irri-tability, sensation, perception, impulse emotions, and symbols and a grandiose, narcissistic,

and concrete sense of self, generally referred to as "egoic"). All these are foundational and necessary for growth into the next stage, the personal, which is associated with the middle stages of social collectives (early state/empire, nation/state) and organization (agrarian, industrial, informational), cultural (mythic, rational, androgynous), behavioral (neocortex, complex neocortex), and consciousness (concepts, rules, formal logic). Balanced preper-sonal and personal development, at least including the four basic lines within the four quadrants of the human holon, are pre-requisites for transpersonal stage development but not for the experiencing of transpersonal *states,* which are available to children, crimi-nals, accident victims, and those who almost die. Transpersonal states are temporary and notoriously difficult to replicate. People who have them can be so impressed that they often conclude that they are enlightened, that is, stabilized at some transpersonal stage of development.

"Transpersonal" refers not only experiences of oneness or unity with nature (nature or "energic" mysticism, the "path of the yogis"), with deity (devotional or love-based mysticism, the "path of the saints"), with formlessness (empty or witnessing mysticism, the "path of the sages") and the non-dual (integration of the secular and sacred). For a discipline to be "transpersonal," it has to do more than provide temporary state openings into oneness, since these are available at any and every stage of development; it has to provide ongoing access to levels of development that transcend the self. All yogas claim to access the transpersonal, but that may only mean they provide temporary state openings; verification of stable stage access to transpersonal perspectives is a matter of following an empirical, injunctive method which involves following instructions and having results verified by peers in the methodology.

These principles are what makes a practice *integal* and transpersonal, according to IDL, and is based on the AQAL model of Ken Wilber. The following diagram is taken from Wilber, K. (1995). *Sex, Ecology, Spirituality, The Spirit of Evolution.* Boston: Shambala.

2   These principles are what makes a practice *integal* and transpersonal, according to IDL, and is based on the AQAL model of Ken Wilber. See the four-quadrant diagram which originally appeared in Wilber, K. (1995). *Sex, Ecology, Spirituality: The Spirit of Evolution.* Boston: Shambala: www.kheper.net/topics/Wilber/Wilber_IV.html

Bibliography

Moreno, J. L. (1934). *Who shall survive? A new approach to the problem of human interrelations.* Boston, MA: Beacon House.

Wilber, K. (1995). *Sex, ecology, spirituality, The spirit of evolution.* Boston: Shambala.

Chapter 3

The origins of Dream Sociometry

Genius ... means little more than the faculty of perceiving in an unhabitual way.

William James[1]

Sociometry defined

J. L. Moreno certainly met James's definition of genius. The creator of psycho-drama and coiner of the term "group psychotherapy" was brilliantly creative. A psychiatrist by training and a younger contemporary of Freud's, Moreno coined the term "Sociometry" in 1918. It means "*the measurement of social groups.*" Moreno also defined sociometry as, "*the mathematical study of psychological properties of populations.*"[2] Any methodology that concerns itself with the nature and measurement of group structures and processes owes a significant debt to Moreno's work. Because Dream Sociometry, the foundational method-ology of IDL, is largely derived from Moreno, it will be helpful to take a brief look at Moreno's sociometry and some of its applications.

Moreno's transpersonal/philosophical orientation

Moreno studied philosophy at the University of Vienna before going on to receive his M.D. from the University of Vienna Medical School in 1917. Fun-damental to Moreno's approach was a profound belief in man's transpersonal nature. His earliest writings are religious and philosophical. He believed that this nature was best expressed through spontaneous action and interaction. Moreno aspired to a religion based upon acknowledging God's attributes in each person, emphasizing the capacity to bring out the creator in every person.

> It is interesting to note that Moreno's ideas about creativity and spontaneity were first reflected in his poetic and theological works, which were written before he ever developed the psychodramatic method as a psychotherapeutic technique. Moreno's writings about the dynamic encounter between man and God in a co-creative rela-tionship take on new relevance today.[3]

The origins of Dream Sociometry

Spontaneity and creativity – concepts fundamental to Moreno

> *As it must not, so genius cannot be lawless; for it is even this that constitutes its genius – the power of acting creatively under laws of its own origination.*
>
> Samuel Taylor Coleridge

For Moreno, creativity and spontaneity impress the very roots of vitality and transpersonal development, thereby influencing every aspect of life. His therapeutic methods consequently emphasize the encouragement of spontaneous expression and the clarification of interactional dynamics within a context of love and mutual sharing. Psychodrama, which Moreno created in 1921 out of earlier explorations he conducted into group psychotherapy, sociometry, and improvisational theater, is most illustrative of the first of these factors. Moreno's sociometry is most illustrative of the second.[4]

Major characteristics of Moreno's underlying approach include "encounter," hermeneutics, phenomenology, existentialism, social constructivism, and postmodernism. All of these strands can be observed within IDL and Dream Sociometry, in the form of encounter with multiple perspectives, whether derived from subjective or objective realms; interpretation, but with the difference that these are primarily made not by the subject, teachers, therapists, or external others, but by interviewed emerging potentials; and existentialism, but with emphasis on meaning as defined by multiple interviewed perspectives rather than the subject, not social constructivism, or the development of knowledge through one's own efforts through interaction with others and their ideas, but *intrasocial constructivism*, in which emphasis is placed on interaction with the ideas and assumed perspectives of dream characters and the personifications of life issues. Postmodernism emphasizes the contextual nature of experience, which condition the possibilities, conclusions, and behaviors that are perceived and activated. In Dream Sociometry, the intrasocial context provides multiple sub-contexts, as defined by the world views and perceptual cognitive distortions of whatever characters are interviewed. This provides radically different contexts which in turn may provide radically different and even transformational possibilities, conclusions, and behaviors.

Why Moreno developed sociometry

Moreno understood that it is possible to gain insight into individual behavior by studying group behavior. Individuals within a group interact and these interactions form patterns of behavior, what Moreno termed each individual's "cultural conserve." Sociometry was developed to provide a framework for exploring the involvement of interactional elements in the development of each person's cultural conserve. This was significant for Moreno because he recognized that what has been learned in action and interaction with others as a child may also be unlearned in action and interaction with others later in life.

Moreno believed that the nature and relationship of these group processes are not always evident and are not always what they seem. While certain aspects of group functioning are overt, others are not readily observable. Moreno recognized that such covert factors – needs, thoughts, purposes, and feelings – are at least as important to group productivity and cohesiveness as are the more obvious aspects of group performance – work output, time allotment, and environmental elements. Moreno developed his sociometric method as a way to gather reliable data about covert group processes. With an increased comprehension of these factors, he believed it would be possible to better understand patterns of group interaction. Analysis of sociometric information could then be used to 1) restructure a group, 2) improve its ability to attain its goals, and 3) increase each group member's degree of satisfaction and productivity. Moreno believed that

> *Scientific foundations of group psychotherapy require as a prerequisite a basic science of human relations, widely known as sociometry. It is from "sociatry," a pathological counterpart of such a science, that knowledge can be derived as to abnormal organization of groups, the diagnosis and prognosis, prophylaxi and control of deviate group behavior.*[5]

Some of the goals of Moreno's sociometry include:

Facilitate constructive change in individuals and groups.
Increase awareness, empathy, reciprocity, and social interactions.
Explore social choice patterns and reduce conflicts.
Clarify roles, interpersonal relations, and values.
Reveal overt and covert group dynamics.
Increase group cohesion and productivity.[6]

Moreno's basic method

Moreno discovered that he could detect covert patterns of group functioning by questioning the members of groups. He would first identify a problem, such as the number of runaways occurring at a girl's reform school. Moreno would then ask the girls questions he called "sociometric tests." For example, one such question would be, "*Who would you most like to have as a roommate?*" The answers to such a question expressed students' preferences toward their schoolmates. These perspective-revealing responses Moreno called "sociometric preferences." Such preferences are simply choices: they can be either positive or negative. In every study, all group members are asked the same questions. Their responses are then tabulated in a grid, called a *sociomatrix*.

Elicitation of sociometric preferences

This method made it possible for Moreno to determine numerically which group members were chosen most often, which were chosen least often, which formed sub-groups or cliques and which were most separated from the rest. The resulting information could then be expressed visually in a diagram called a *sociogram*, in which covert patterns of relationship and interaction among the members of a group become overt. In the application of sociometric procedures mentioned above, the behavioral patterns of girls in a reform school were restructured in a way that significantly reduced the incidence of runaways.

Moreno's impact

> *We are accustomed to see men deride what they do not understand and snarl at the good and beautiful because it lies beyond their sympathies.*
>
> Johann Wolfgang Von Goethe

In the later years of his life, Moreno felt that his work had been largely ignored by the mainstream of psychology and sociology, a fact about which he felt some bitterness. Moreno's innovations in group psychotherapy predated and stimulated much good work in both psychology and sociology. In fact, his action methods were not ignored; his methods were widely appropriated, largely without attribution, appropriate recognition of their source, or appreciation of the philosophical context in which they were embedded.

This was partially because Moreno's basic assumptions about psychology and experimental method sprang from a different world view than the prevailing scientific humanistic, positivist *zeitgeist*. Moreno believed in a spontaneous, subjective approach to knowledge and to life, which he saw springing from an essentially transpersonal reality. Consequently, more empirically based contemporaries, interested in advancing their field as a recognized science, could appreciate and borrow specific techniques and methods advocated by Moreno while having little in common with the perceptual framework from which they sprouted.

For example, psychiatrist Fritz Perls, developer of Gestalt therapy, was strongly affected by Moreno's psychodrama in the development of his role-playing techniques.

> *In fact, Fritz Perls, founder of Gestalt therapy, admitted to the author of this work that he had taken most of his ideas directly from Moreno's work. It is unfortunate that in so adapting his techniques, many practitioners, teachers and writers in the*

field have failed to acknowledge Dr. Moreno's innovations and contributions. It is perhaps even more unfortunate that in the popularization of these psychodramatic techniques, the profound and creative philosophy behind Dr. Moreno's work has rarely been considered.[7]

Psychiatrist Eric Berne, the creator of Transactional Analysis, wrote:

In his selection of specific techniques, Dr. Perls shares with other 'active' psychothera-pists the "Moreno problem": That nearly all known "active" techniques were first tried out by Dr. J.L. Moreno in psychodrama, so that it is difficult to come up with an original idea in this regard.[8]

A. H. Maslow wrote,

I would however like to add one credit-where-credit-is-due footnote. Many of the techniques set forth in the article (dealing with encounter techniques) were originally invented by Dr. Jacob Moreno, who is still functioning vigorously and probably still inventing new techniques and ideas.[9]

Dr. William Schutz (a major figure in the encounter group movement) noted that,

Virtually all of the methods that I had proudly compiled or invented {Moreno} had more or less anticipated, in some cases forty years earlier . . . Leuner's original article (on guided fantasy) has appeared in (Moreno's) Journal in about 1932 and he had been using the method periodically since . . . I invite you to investigate Moreno's work. It is probably not sufficiently acknowledged in this country. Perl's Gestalt Therapy owes a great deal to it. It is imaginative and worth exploring.[10]

It was primarily Moreno's emphasis on spontaneity, creativity, and the transper-sonal that caused Moreno to be ignored by the majority of his intellectual contemporaries. They liked his methods but had little understanding of the perspective from which they sprang. The fields of psychiatry and psychology were, in the first half of the 20th century, striving mightily to prove that they were empirically based sciences, and Moreno's theories, methods, and tempera-ment were not in step with the prevailing mental health *zeitgeist*. In terms of the perennial philosophy, the prevailing world view was rationalistic. Reason was king. Moreno's advocacy of spontaneity, creativity, and the transpersonal looked like a prepersonal throwback from the perspective of contemporaries instead of the early transpersonal structure that it actually presented. In this regard, Moreno met the same fate that Wilber's integral was to meet at the hands of the American Psychological Association in the 1990's, when they decided it was too "spiritual" for formal inclusion in the field of psychology.

Applications of Moreno's sociometry

Since the 1930s, Moreno's sociometric techniques have been used in military, business, mental health, social service, and political applications.

In its business applications, sociometry has been used to identify accident-prone people, reduce absenteeism, reduce breakage in factories, and even help resolve executive kidnappings. Conflicts between management and labor, older and younger workers, and between workers in different departments have all been reduced through the use of sociometry. Reduction of conflicts among members of secretarial pools has been achieved, and sociometrically based accounting procedures have been developed.

The military has used sociometry to reduce sick call incidence, to predict which bomber crews would be least likely to return from sorties, and to plan personnel and ship deployment. Browne (1951) used a sociometry-like questionnaire to study the relationships among a group of 24 executives. The data were used to graphically depict 1) the formal organization of the company and 2) interaction patterns among the executives. Further analysis of the data on a divisional basis revealed marked differences in the relations existing between the executives in these units. How frequently an executive interacted with others seemed to be correlated with responsibility, authority, and delegation of authority.[11]

In the field of education, sociometry has been used to promote learning by providing a favorable environment for group interaction. Sociometry can predict which students are most likely to drop out of school. It has also been used to improve individual student study habits and performance. Pollsters have used sociometry to help predict national and local election results.

Rogers (1946) studied human problems in industry and was convinced that the most significant contributions to the understanding of the psychological problems of workers has been made by J. L. Moreno in the form of sociometric measures and, secondly, the Harvard Business School group. Van Zelst (1952) indicates that for industrial success in using sociometry, it is essential that management 1) have a democratic approach to its workers and 2) recognize the importance of group relations and manifest and interest in work preferences. Interestingly, these same factors are vital if a dreamer is to understand and support greater internal integration through the use of Dream Sociometry.

There are many reasons to believe that sociometry is a useful tool with many undiscovered applications in a variety of fields. As more individuals are exposed to techniques of behavioral self-change, control of growth is being transferred from the hands of specialists and placed in the sphere of the patient or subject, with the therapist becoming a facilitator of this process. Moreno would have heartily approved of such an evolution in areas he dedicated his life to nourishing. More information about sociometric applications may be found in the journal *Sociometry*.

Summary

- In 1917, J. L. Moreno invented Sociometry, a method of revealing and assessing the covert preferences of members of groups.
- While sometimes not attributed to Moreno, his methods have been applied in military, business, mental health, social service, and political applications.
- IDL is an elaboration based on Dream Sociometry, a direct descendant of Moreno's sociometric methods.

Notes

1 James, W. (1890). *The Principles of Psychology*.
2 Moreno, J. L. (1934). *Who Shall Survive? A new Approach to the Problem of Human Interrelations*. Boston, MA: Beacon House, p. 33.
3 Blatner, A. (1973). *Acting in*. New York: Springer.
4 Blatner, *Acting in*, foreword.
5 Moreno, J. L. (1953). *Who Shall Survive? Foundations of Sociometry, Group Psychotherapy and Sociodrama*. Boston, MA: Beacon House.
6 Sociometry. *American Society of Group Therapy and Psychodrama*. www.asgpp.org/soc2.htm
7 Rudhyar, D. (1976). *An Astrological Study of Psychological Complexes*, p. 73.
8 Howie, P. (Summer 2012). *Philosophy of life: J. L. Moreno's revolutionary philosophical underpinnings of psychodrama, and group psychotherapy*. Group: The Journal of the Eastern Group Psychotherapy Society, *36*(2), 135–146.
9 Letter to Editors, *LIFE Magazine*, August 2, 1968.
10 Schulz, W., quoted in Blatner, *Acting in*.
11 Hart, J., & Nath, R. (1979). Sociometry in Business and Industry. *Journal of Group Psychotherapy, Psychodrama and Sociometry*, *32*, 135.

Bibliography

Blatner, A. (1973). *Acting in*. New York: Springer.
Hart, J., & Nath, R. (1979). Sociometry in business and industry. *Journal of Group Psychotherapy, Psychodrama and Sociometry*, *32*, 135.
Howie, P. (2012, Summer). *Philosophy of life: J. L. Moreno's revolutionary philosophical underpinnings of psychodrama, and group psychotherapy*.
Group: The Journal of the Eastern Group Psychotherapy Society, Volume 36.2, pp. 135–146.
James, W. (1890). *The principles of psychology*.
Moreno, J. L. (1953). *Who shall survive? Foundations of sociometry, group psychotherapy and sociodrama*. Boston, MA: Beacon House.
Rudhyar, D. (1976). An Astrological Study of Psychological Complexes. Princeton, NJ, Sociometry, American Society of Group Therapy and Psychodrama.

Chapter 4

Interviewed dream characters and your waking roles

Man cannot discover new oceans unless he has courage to lose sight of the shore.

Andre Gide

Moreno's rules for role players

Moreno offers three simple and relevant guidelines for role players: *Give truth to receive truth. Give love to the group and it will return love to you. Give spontaneity and spontaneity will return.*[1] This is wise guidance for you as you identify with interviewed characters when you create a Dream Sociomatrix. Be truthful in your interactions with those perspectives you interview. Love them. Be spontaneous. Following these guidelines in your applications of Dream Sociometry can only enhance the benefit you will receive from the experience.

The importance of "taking the role of the other"

Imagination is more important than knowledge.

Albert Einstein

Moreno advocated growth through constructive, creative interaction between spontaneous beings. The more passive or "doll"-like an individual is, the slower learning becomes.[2] For sociologist George Herbert Mead, social control and social cohesion depend on man's capacity to be an object to himself and to take the role of the other. Your intrasocial control and cohesion also depend largely upon your ability to be an object to yourself and to take the role of the other. You do this when you identify with your interviewed characters in IDL. Wilber speaks of this in terms of differentiating your "distal" selves from your "proximate" self.

Your dreams work to help maintain your internal psychic homeostasis by naturally providing experiences in which you are an object to yourself and take the role of the other, in the form of the entire dream drama, with all its

characters, objects, and settings. Unfortunately, you rarely relate this autonomous inner process to your waking life in a way that allows you to become a
co-creator in your internal evolution. By *"taking the role of the other"* through
Dream Sociometric element identification, you become an object to yourself.
Your proximate self, your sense of "I," becomes another distal "me," one of the
many roles that you take. Through identification with interviewed characters
you internalize and integrate the inclusive yet transcendent perspectives they
personify. This speeds development, lucidity, clarity, waking up, and, indeed,
enlightenment, by first increasing awareness of crucial blind spots and by then
putting that awareness to work in a practical sort of way.

When you actively involve yourself with your dreams groups, accepting
them on their own terms as a significant reality in and of themselves, you
speed the creativity and the constructive nature of the spontaneous interaction
between the focus of your awareness and its surrounding field. You loosen up.
You become more child-like in your spontaneity; you open your eyes to inner
potentials that you never before recognized.

Waking state identification with interviewed dream characters

There is another important reason why it is very useful to take the role of your
interviewed characters. Many drug studies have shown that if an animal learns
to navigate a maze under the influence of a drug, he may be unable to do so
again until he is again in a drugged state. This phenomenon is called state-
dependent learning. It would follow that if you desire to have a truly meaningful waking relationship with dream reality you might best identify with dream
awareness as closely as possible while you are awake. To fully comprehend a
dream, you need to mimic the state you were in when you experienced it.
Dream Sociometric interviewed character identificationcharacter is one way of
striving to re-create the dream as vividly as possible from as many perspectives
as possible in the context of your waking dream. This theory is validated by the
common experience of remembering forgotten aspects of dreams in the process of becoming and interviewing its characters. Another way you can initiate
a dialogue with dream awareness is by reviewing elicited interviewed character
elaborations and dreamages during the hypnogogic state, when imagery is most
likely to occur naturally and you are most suggestible.

The commonness of taking roles in waking life

You do not have to access an altered state to become a dream character or to
do Dream Sociometry. There is no reason why your normal waking awareness
cannot meaningfully take the perspective of dream elements, since interviewed
characters have a phenomenological existence that is at least partially dependent upon your perceptual assumptions. Interviewed characters are aspects of
contexts that expand as you do, of which your waking awareness remains

merely one limited and partial perspective, although it is itself a composite of many alternating roles. In your waking life, interviewed characters exist as non-personified role expectations, perspectives, and beliefs, some of which you are commonly aware of, but most of which remain in the background of your awareness. Some are clearly mostly aspects of yourself; others are very much non-self. In your dream life, these same elements exercise autonomous existence as subsystems of a broader perceptual matrix which views your waking identity as only one of many valid perspectives on a much more broadly experienced reality.

The importance of role conflict as a source of dream roles

Role conflict is an ongoing and serious issue for all of us because we routinely experience role identification many times throughout the day. We seamlessly "become" consumers, drivers, workers, parents, one after another. It is extremely rare to simultaneously experience ourselves as all of these things at the same time while we are awake, although at any one time we often wear two or more such hats: mother and wife, employee and supervisor, seller and consumer. When you are awake, you rarely notice the inconsistencies between your personality at work and your personality at a party or at church. To imagine yourself acting like you do at a wild party while in church is embarrassing even to contemplate. Perhaps you love your family while you complain about your neighbors; you give to your church and fudge on your taxes; you expect others to keep their commitments and then are chronically late to your appointments. You expect yourself to be loving but find yourself fighting instead; you find self-esteem in your career but are unemployed; you pride yourself on your concern for your employees only to have them unite against you due to your unfairness. You will experience such uncomfortable conflicts among your waking life roles only when you have little choice.

When this occurs, the recognition of role conflicts can create deeply disturbing cognitive dissonance that ripples through both body and mind. Such inconsistencies are associated with less coherent brain wave patterns and may contribute to diminished immunological functioning, imbalanced hormonal secretions, and a resulting host of physical maladies. We therefore disown such role conflicts, if only as a basic survival strategy.

These roles only occur at the same time when they are compatible. Contradictory roles rarely confront us in waking life because we do our utmost to repress, ignore, or deny those inconsistencies. However, when you are dreaming, rules of compatibility that govern waking are suspended. Dream groups commonly present you with these incongruences, routinely confronting you with discrepancies among your various identities. You tolerate them only because your ability to detect and challenge such glaring, embarrassing and awkward role inconsistencies is normally suspended in your dreams.

Because time is much altered when you dream, your roles, personified as different dream characters, come into contact in ways that never happens in waking life. Those roles constellate in dreams which relate to the particular life issues with which the dream deals. You are thereby provided in your dreams with opportunities to recognize how contradictory much of your behavior actually is. For example, if the dream is concerned with how you lose your temper, but normally justify it and ignore it, characters that personify your contradictory perspectives and preferences about impulse control are likely to come together. There may be a fire in a house and maybe a fire truck and another house. Each of these characters, if interviewed, will have its own opinion about the nature, genesis, and solution to your temper outbursts.

Dream opportunities to recognize how contradictory our roles are generally go unrecognized because we lack sufficient lucidity. Dream Sociometry, however, identifies these role contradictions when we are in our waking, relatively lucid state, allowing us to reduce both waking and dream dissonance. This, in turn, creates less conflict in dreams and moves into greater dream lucidity.

Summary

- Role identification is a normal occurrence in both development and daily life. We are always in one or more roles.
- Consequently, role identification is neither difficult nor unusual.
- Because our conflicting waking roles are normally separated by time and context, conflict among roles generates unrecognized dissonance.
- Dreaming normally brings contradictory roles into contact, but because our rational faculties are suspended, we miss opportunities to recognize these inconsistencies and do something about them.
- Dream Sociometry confronts us with our role inconsistencies in ways that not only brings them to our attention but allows us to take steps to reduce the cognitive dissonance they can create.
- When you witness yourself from alternative perspectives, you relativize your identity and your perspective. This expands your identity to incorporate other perspectives.
- Consequently, the act of role identification itself cultivates objectivity and witnessing.
- Character role identification in Dream Sociometry identifies and reduces both internal and social conflict.

Notes

1 Moreno, J. L. (1934). *Who Shall Survive?* p. 114.
2 Moreno, J. L. (1934). *Who Shall Survive?* p. 68.

Bibliography

Moreno, J. L. (1934). *Who shall survive? A new approach to the problem of human interrelations.* Boston, MA: Beacon House.

Chapter 5

Enhancing dream recall

Emphasize quality over quantity

It is common to assume that dreamwork requires remembering and writing down many dreams. The good news is that you need not recall many of your dreams in order to derive transformative results from your dreamwork. As a matter of fact, Dream Sociometry can be effectively applied to waking events, which are, after all, subject to the same foibles of individual perception that we bring to dreams. When we appreciate that life is a dream and dreams are life, without in any way diminishing the reality of either, we realize that we have material for productive interviewing available to us at all times, whether or not we remember our dreams.

Because life transformation is based on daily application rather than insight, IDL emphasizes the *quality* of your application of Action Plans derived from the recommendations of those emerging potentials that you interview. Consequently, while dream recall is a helpful form of cybernetic feedback to speed your awakening, it is not essential to learning and applying Dream Sociometry or using IDL. This is important for people who remember few dreams, such as those who have sustained a brain injury or whose attention is simply directed elsewhere.

However, few people have difficulty remembering enough dreams to keep them well supplied for the creation of Dream Sociomatrices, since only one or two a month are quite sufficient for all but the most hard-core transpersonal explorers. Because of the in-depth focus you give to each dream or life situation when you create a Dream Sociomatrix, there tends to arise an increasing congruence between your waking and your internal agendas. Consequently, you may find your recall improving. Since you are no longer going your own way, oblivious to the priorities of life, your motivation to suppress your dreams recedes. On the other hand, you may find that as you practice integral deep listening you wake up out of drama, and, as a result, the emotional intensity of your dreams subsides. Consequently, you may find that you are less likely to spontaneously remember them. This is because you are listening to, respecting, and acting on factors that generated the internal conflicts that created drama and emotional intensity in your life. Therefore, you may find that you need to focus your intent to recall dreams as you become increasingly healthy and balanced.

Now, having hopefully lowered any pressure you may be putting on yourself to remember a lot of dreams, there remain reasons why you might want to increase your recall. There are also any number of strategies that can help you enhance your dream recall.

To increase recall, increase your awareness of your dreams

As Erving Goffman has pointed out, we treat our dreams as if they were mental patients:

> In a psychiatric hospital, failure to be an easily manageable patient – failure, for example, to work or to be polite to the staff – tends to be taken as evidence that one is not yet "ready" for liberty and that one has need of further treatment. The point is not that the hospital is a hateful place for patients, but that for the patient to express hatred of it is to give evidence that his place in it is justified and that he is not yet ready to leave it.

Similarly, when we have "bad dreams," our first reaction is often to repress our dreams. We relegate parts of ourselves to the dungeons and our internal psych wards, generally because triviality, absurdity, fear, shame, and a sense of threat to our image of ourselves are powerful forces that encourage us to dismiss almost all of our dreams. Then we are free to continue to run our lives as we like, following our unilateral waking agenda, without taking into account questioning, dissenting perspectives. While comfortable and common, such dismissal is also dangerous, if not deadly. At the very least, it leads to decreased self-awareness until our issues become so intense that they will no longer be ignored. They may then externalize as the waking nightmares of disease, accident, or a dysfunctional life.

Dream recall can be enhanced by strengthening attributes in each of the four quadrants of the human holon. From the perspective of the individual internal quadrant that addresses thoughts, feelings, and level of development, dream recall is primarily a function of intent. Increase your desire to remember your dreams, and you are likely to recall them. Increase your awareness of your dreams, and you automatically increase your dream recall. Attention is another internal individual aspect of dream recall. Most non-recallers wake up some minutes after their last dream sequence has been completed, while recallers wake up just as their dream concludes. They forget to pay attention to their dreams and instead immediately begin to think about what they have to do in the coming day. You reduce your awareness of your dreams when you take stimulants, depressants, get caught up in an overwhelmingly external life focus, or simply through self-indulgence. These are individual *external* blocks to dream recall and reflect individual exterior holon barriers.

You can practice Dream Sociometry and IDL without ever remembering a dream. For instance, if you have had a brain injury and your ability to recall dreams is impaired, you can work with emotions, life events, and images from guided fantasy. If you have difficulty remembering any dreams at all, begin by working with a life issue or story that reflects a repetitive source of fear, failure, rejection, abandonment, sadness, abandonment, or loneliness. You can also work with dream from your past, preferably a dream that you have had more than once. If you remember only one dream and it occurred when you were five, start there. Work with it! By priming the pump, you will increase your intent, awareness, and attention.

Use simple pre-sleep suggestion

Giving yourself pre-sleep suggestions is an excellent way to increase your awareness of your dreams. For instance, you can repeat, "*I will remember my dreams when I awaken in the morning.*" Such suggestions, which are meanings and values representative of the internal collective quadrant of the human holon, focus your intent. They encourage you to turn your attention to your dreams upon awakening and increase the likelihood that you will awaken immediately after a dream cycle has been completed, when you are most likely to remember your dreams.

Those that have difficulty with such suggestions are usually in conflict about maintaining the internal vigilance that is required to be aware that they are dreaming, since this is in conflict with another goal – to sleep as soundly as possible. Many people carry an inbred sense that dream recall is an enemy of sound, comfortable sleep.

Tips for enhancing recall

If you do not remember your dreams or run into a dry spell, here are some suggestions to improve your dream recall.

- As stated above, suggest to yourself before going to sleep that you will remember your dreams.
- As you drift off to sleep, visualize yourself waking up and remembering a dream. See yourself reaching for your pen and note card and writing the dream. An example of such a pre-sleep suggestion is, "*I am now asleep and it is just before I will awaken to start my day. I'm dreaming and I know that I want to remember this dream when I awaken. I am now awakening as the dream concludes. I am pleased with the clarity of my recall of the dream. I am now reaching for my pen and clipboard. I turn on the light and as I begin to write, my dreams come flooding back in satisfying completeness. I feel rested, exhilarated and very pleased.*"

- Tell yourself that crazy, scary, and confusing dreams that make no sense to you and appear worthless are as valuable as divine revelations; you just don't have the perspective or understanding to recognize it. However, you know that you can develop it by practicing Dream Sociometry with such dreams.
- Visualize yourself awakening alert and refreshed. This will tend to counteract fear that dream recall is going to reduce the quality of your sleep.
- Stress increases dream recall, particularly emotional agitation and turmoil. While distress is to be avoided, eustress, or healthy stress, can be cultivated as a way of increasing dream recall. Strong feelings of helpfulness, thankfulness, personal satisfaction, or joy are likely to increase your dream recall, as are anticipation for what you will learn or events of the next day.
- Meditation clarifies and focuses attention and has been shown to improve dream recall, dream coherence and the perceived helpfulness of dreams. Meditation before sleep will tend to reduce your emotional conflicts from the day, making it less likely that they will induce physiologically stressful dreams. This is another internal individual approach to increasing dream recall, in that it clarifies consciousness itself, thereby eliminating barriers to experiences of all kinds.
- Look over your dreams before you go to sleep. Bedtime dream review stimulates interest, awareness, and intent, improving recall.
- Read about dreams, dreaming, lucid dreaming, or related topics before you go to sleep.
- Apply in your daily life those dreams that you do choose to work with. Dream application improves recall. This approach to dream recall utilizes the external individual and collective quadrants of the human holon. Taking dreams seriously and working with them in your daily life should improve both the quantity and the quality of your dreams.
- If you do not remember a dream when you awaken, ask yourself, "How do I feel?" Name your feeling. Are you happy? Are you sad? Confused? Irritated? Anxious? Self-critical? Strengthen your awareness of that feeling; doing so will often trigger a flood of dream images.
- Make sure you get your minimum daily requirement of the B vitamins. A deficiency can impair dream recall.
- Barbiturates and amphetamines decrease dream sleep. Sleeping pills, coffee, caffeinated drinks, alcohol, and tranquilizers interfere with dream recall. Don't take them before bed if you want to remember your dreams. Hallucinogens also create problems with dream recall.
- Again, remember that *quality* of recall is more important than *quantity*. Do a thorough job of understanding and applying those dreams you do remember, and you will be ahead of the person who remembers many, many dreams.
- Explore any feelings of resistance to recall you may have in writing or discuss it with a friend. Give it a color, then an expanse, then a shape. Interview the shape regarding the nature, source, and solution to the resistance using the IDL life issue protocol.

- Join an IDL Sangha or Integral Salon or create your own. Sharing and discussing dreams is a powerful external collective way of increasing dream recall.
- If you have been working with IDL, you can interview previously interviewed emerging potentials regarding what you can do to increase dream recall. This is an internal collective approach to increasing your dream recall.

Summary

- An in-depth interview every now and then is much superior to great recall and a superficial relationship with your emerging potentials.
- Understanding common blockages and resistances to dream recall will help you to evaluate your priorities honestly. Do you really want to recall your dreams?
- If you decide that you want to increase your dream recall, there are many different strategies that have been found to be helpful for many people. Experiment until you find a combination that works for you.

Chapter 6

Recording your dreams

Everything secret degenerates; nothing is safe that does not bear discussion and publicity.
Lord Acton

General considerations choosing which dream to work with

Those who argue against dreamwork on the grounds that it disturbs a natural order better left to its own devices merely cut themselves off from inner well-springs of creativity as well as a powerful tool for the cultivation of equanimity. While working with dreams is optional with IDL, it teaches a growing respect for inner wisdom, acceptance, empathy, peace, witnessing, and confidence that transcends that possessed by waking identity. As you proceed in your understanding of IDL, your choice of dreams to work with may also change. At first, many wisely choose dreams that contain repeating themes. By doing so these themes throw light on many related dreams that are not evaluated in depth. Initially, choose dreams that interest you. These could be nightmares from your childhood, psychic experiences, or inspirational visions full of archetypes. As you progress, you may find that you gain the most from listening to those dreams that *don't* interest you. This is because our waking agenda is not a reliable guide to understanding the priorities of our life compass. Laying our waking preferences aside and just going with a typical recalled dream is often highly enlightening.

Be prepared!

Good dreamwork habits save time and energy while supporting quality contact with your dreams. Be prepared to catch a wild dream as it floats by! Keep a small light (bedside or flashlight) and some way of capturing your dreams by your bed, such as pencil and paper, tape recorder, or computer. When you awaken, think about your feelings before moving. When you are satisfied that your dreams are clear in your thinking, begin writing. Sometimes you will remember more of your dream as you begin to write.

Ways of recording dreams

Until the day we can just plug ourselves in at night and watch the video play-back in the morning, recall will continue to require some vigilance. Fortunately, there are almost as many ways to record dreams as there are individual styles. Some people use a diary, others a tape recorder. I now have students who use voice-activated computer dictation, which is a spectacular new technology. I look forward to the day when the entire Dream Sociometric interviewing and tabulation process is voice activated and both Dream Sociomatrix and Dream Sociogram are automatically created.[1] For years, I preferred the low-tech use of lined note cards for recording and storing dreams. I then transcribed them in chronological order into yearly dream and dreamwork files and kept the originals in note-card boxes for chronological archiving. For almost 20 years now, I have just typed them into my computer. While the following instructions assume writing, because it is always nice to be able to continue your inner work if you do not have access to artificial brains, use whatever method works best for you.

Write the dream or life experience in 1st-person, present tense

For example: "*I am a snake charmer watching a cobra rise out of its basket over the end of my flute.*" Stick to what happened when you write down a dream account. Include all feelings, using such words as angry, thankful, confused, guilty, happy, scared, upset, and sad. Record not only your feelings, but also any implied by the behavior or words of other dream characters. This will help you to "get back" into the dream when you begin to work on it, re-experiencing it in the 1st-person present tense. At that time, see all the colors and places. Feel the emotions of the dream once again. Re-create it! This will help to clarify and intensify the statement of preferences by different interviewed characters. Leave your associations for the section that follows your dream or life experience account.

Dating and numbering dreams

If you do voice dictation or type them up on your computer, be sure and include the date. If you use Dream Sociometry with more than one dream from a night, it is helpful to have them numbered. Write down dream fragments; you will find that IDL works just as well with dream fragments as it does for an entire dream.

Give your dream a title

A title that captures and communicates a major theme of your experience will help you to quickly recall the entire dream and to find it again quickly when you need it. To create a title, ask yourself, "*If this dream were to appear as a book or a movie, what would the best title for it be?*" A good name will convey both the action and the feeling of the dream. Sometimes a simple name is sufficient, such as "*The giant squid.*" More often, verbs or noun clauses do the trick, as in "*Running Scared,*" or "*The Helpless Hero.*" Titles personalize dreams, make their content easier to recall, and help you begin your dialogue with your creation.

Here is an example of a dream that we will refer through as we move through this text:

Ken Wilber Dies 08/27/01 Joseph Dillard
I hear that Ken Wilber and his girlfriend are killed in a head-on car crash.
   I am upset.

Note associations to your daily life

After you have finished writing down the dream, note any associations that come to mind. A few short phrases will do. Ask yourself, "*What does this experience remind me of? Do any of the events relate to recent waking happenings? Do the interviewed characters remind me of any people I know in real life?*" Write something in the association section, even if it is "No idea!" Associations anchor the event at a certain historical point in your life. They also create a sort of a pre-test. It is not unusual for a dreamer to feel, after they have listened to the interviewed characters in their dream, that they "knew that all along!" Since your dream images are personifications of perspectives, it is not surprising that on some level, you already know whatever comes out of your dreamwork. On the other hand, if you already knew it, why didn't you say so in your associations before you worked on the dream? Your associations give you a sense of those awarenesses that were more or less obvious to you before you started listening to your interviewed characters. What comes out of your interviewing is not necessarily novel information, since you already know truths about your life on some level of awareness, but rather a difference in emphasis or priority. You are stuck not so much because of what you don't know, but because of the way you prioritize what you do know.[2] Your priorities are, for one reason or another, not transformative.[3] IDL aligns your priorities with those of your life compass. Noting your associations and then going back and reviewing them is one way of convincing yourself that real and fundamental change is happening.

The Associations to *Ken Wilber Dies* are:

> *My associations to this dream are* . . . I greatly respect Ken Wilber and look forward not only to his next book, but am excited about the way he is influencing authorities in many different fields. For him to die in a car crash sounds like a warning that I am doing something to kill the parts of myself which he represents – clear, objective, personally dedicated to transpersonal development and supporting others to do the same.

Criteria for choosing a dream to work on

You will not create a Dream Sociomatrix for every dream you remember, nor will you need to. To learn how your preferences both support and hinder your development you do not need to deeply listen to all perspectives all the time. The reality is that you are only centrally stuck in a few critical places or areas, and your preferences, as well as the conflicts they disclose, will return again and again to them. Therefore, overcoming dysfunction and getting unstuck is not a bottomless pit. Most fears dissolve when listened to; they do not give away to an endless regression to into deeper realms of Dante's *Inferno*. Quality identification with only a few emerging potentials at appropriate moments can leverage your entire development. This is a core truth of IDL, and I have seen it in action many times. There is good reason to be confident that you will, too.

You can apply this method to any dream or life experience that you choose. Emotions, however, such as fear itself, physical pain, depression, and anger can be directly addressed effectively with the single-character interviewing protocol. Ask yourself the following questions about a dream you are considering working with:

1) "Is the dream of *reasonable length?*"

   How long a dream is it best to work with? Dream Sociometry works best with short dream narratives, with self-contained episodes in longer dreams, or with the high points of longer ones. Start with something short, say a dream or dream scene that will fit on the front of one note card and which contains no more than four nouns (characters, places, and objects), four actions, and four feelings. In fact, you will find that dreams or scripted life issues that contain four nouns will often contain no more than two actions and two feelings. Notice that I picked as an example a dream that can be expressed in one sentence. After you learn the method, you can work with longer dreams, as you will be picking out representative elements to put in the Dream Sociomatrix.

2) "Is the dream fairly *simple in structure?*"

   While learning the process, pick a dream or dream segment that does not have more than 12 elements (characters, actions, and feelings) in total. If you dream only in epics, then work with a distinct dream scene or segment. Interview no more than three characters, in addition to Dream Self and Dream Consciousness, the first time you attempt the process.

3) "Does the dream *interest* me?"

   Does it concern, disturb, puzzle, or otherwise beckon you? After you learn the process, you may well find yourself intrigued by the fact that some dreams don't interest you, and you want to find out why. It will definitely be worth your while to do Dream Sociometry with dreams that do not interest you. However, until you have learned the method, stick with those that intrigue you.

4)   "Have I had this dream *more than once*?"

Repetitive dreams tend to be more important because they address ongoing, repetitive life issues. If you don't remember one, consider creating a story around a repetitive life issue that has been a persistent thorn in your side, and create a Dream Sociomatrix based on it. IDL quickly eliminates most repetitive dreams. You will find that dream themes and patterns generally repeat, making every dream repetitive in several ways.

If you have a sense that a dream is important or relates to a major concern of yours but violates most of these guidelines, go ahead and use it. It may, however, complicate your learning process. For instance, if your dream has more than two scenes in it or contains scenes of some length, you will find you need to work with a shorter piece with fewer elements. Otherwise, you may be creating Dream Sociomatrices that run off your desk and across the floor – not very practical! Later, when you are comfortable with the process, you can choose selected elements from long dreams to place in the Dream Sociomatrix. Do not be overly ambitious until you have mastered the basic methodology or you may burn yourself out before you get started!

Why "old" dreams are still valuable to work with

> *God offers every mind a choice between truth and repose. Take which you please – you can never have both.*
>
> Ralph Waldo Emerson

If you do not get to a dream in a day, a week, a month, or a year, is there any point in still completing the Dream Sociomatrix and the commentaries? Yes, there most definitely is. Dream memories from when you were six still contain relevant and highly useful information for your present life. This is because the characters that you interview will voice perspectives that are *current*; you will hear perspectives that are relevant to your life now, regardless of when you had the dream. The perspectives you access, as well as your comparison of their explanations of their preferences in the various elaborations, will also help you to understand why you approached life as you did at the time that you had the dream – the choices you made, the feelings you had, the problem-solving approaches you used, the actions you pursued. All of this is generally experienced as healing and transformative.

Your dreams deal with your present life

You can never completely re-experience a dream. Even a vivid reliving of a dream or life event is filtered through the context of your present awareness.

Just because you believe you understand why you had a dream or life event provides no assurance that you have accurately resuscitated the past. This is because you can never know for sure what your preferences were at the time you had the dream. All dreamwork is *present tense*; you cannot re-create the past, only enliven the present. You can re-frame your memories in a way that resolve conflict and integrate them as important, supportive components of who you are today. This does not mean, however, that you have recovered the "true" or "actual" reality of what you experienced in the past.

While IDL primarily provides you with understanding about your *present* preferences and state of awareness, since aspects of your awareness repeat over time and stay relatively stable, it is possible to *infer* past relationships from your dreamwork. It is common to change long-standing life patterns that are associated with earlier years. This is a predicament that historical studies of any type find themselves confronting – we think we are talking about the past, but we can only change in the present, including our memories of the past. Remember that you are always primarily talking about *yourself*, not your dreams, as they belong to a reality that transcends but includes you and about *this moment*, not about a past experience such as a dream. This will keep you from making claims for your dreams that are difficult, if not impossible, to substantiate. If you think you already understand a dream completely, you may be surprised at what you discover when you look at it from intrasocial perspectives, as you do with IDL. This is even the case with the nightmares of post-traumatic stress syndrome, which are a vivid reliving of concrete, historical events. When these experiences are relived from the perspectives of objects, characters, and antagonists, awareness often shifts.

When to work on your dream

Is it important *when* you start to work on your dream? While this does not seem to be a major issue, the psychological need to work on a dream while it is still "fresh" is undeniable and a real preference for many people. Most people find IDL is effective in working with dreams they had years before. While you are learning Dream Sociometry it is wise to work on a dream within the week that you recall it. Your associations to your waking life will be clearer, which means that it will be easier for you to recognize the relevance to your current life of what you discover from Dream Sociometry. While current associations are not essential to IDL, they will help you to anchor your dream to waking events, which, in turn, will help you to recognize recurring life patterns, of which a waking association is only one specific instance. With a shorter passage of time, you will have changed less since you had the dream. Consequently, your interviewed character preferences are more likely to reflect actual perspectives held at the time you had the dream. If you work on a dream today you receive information that is relevant to today, not 20 years ago.

When the time does come to work on your dream, expect to spend approximately two to three hours per dream, whether at one sitting or broken up into several. This is because you are interviewing more characters regarding many more of their preferences than you do in the single-character dream or life issue protocols, thereby receiving a much more thorough understanding of why the group precipitated into the constellation that it did. Dream Sociometric, single dream, and life issue protocol templates are available to be copied at DreamYoga.com and also in the appendices. Templates guide you through the structured interviewing of your interviewed characters. To begin, write or cut and paste the dream name, the date you had the dream, your name, the dream narrative, and, finally, any associations that you wrote at the time you recalled the dream or life issue.

Identifying three life issues

How relevant is IDL and Dream Sociometry to the concerns that concerns you the most? What impact does it have on those concerns that matter the most to you? Identifying three life issues is another way of putting IDL to the test. Does it produce help that you can translate into improvements in areas that are of central importance to you? The answers that your interviewed characters give to these concerns in the Waking Commentary will help you decide for yourself how relevant Dream Sociometry and IDL are to those issues that are most important to you.

Here are some examples of some life issues: money, problems with a partner, stress, weight loss, improving your meditation, procrastination, shyness, solving a problem at work. If you choose, you may write them as questions that you would like to have answered. Here are some examples:

Why am I having so much trouble finding a partner?
What do I need to do to get my work team on track with this new assignment?

My mind keeps going when I try to meditate. Any suggestions?
I am always late! What can I do?
I am having trouble keeping my office organized. Help!

Here are examples of three life issues from *Ken Wilber Dies:*

- Am I killing parts of myself that are like Ken Wilber?
- How can I improve my meditation?
- How can I discipline myself to lose this last 15 pounds?

The life issue questions

Two optional questions can follow the life issues, to ask yourself if you like. They are:

If I could resolve these issues, what difference would it make in my life?
What do I think I need to do to be happy in my life?

Their purpose is to define an ideal or "target" state that you are aiming for at the outset of your interviewing process. These questions attempt to make your overt motivations covert so that they can be evaluated and revised as needed, in the light of the information produced by IDL.

Here are these two questions and their answers as they appear in *Ken Wilber Dies*:

If I could resolve these issues, what difference would it make in my life?

I could help more people understand how they sabotage their transpersonal development and what they can do to stop it.

I could help more people meditate better. I would feel less hypocritical and more authentic about practicing what I'm preaching.

I could help other people stick to and attain challenging personal goals. It would increase my self-esteem and get one more irritation out of my life.

What do I think I need to do to be happy in my life?

Listen to myself and demonstrate that I respect myself by acting on the good I hear by making changes in my waking life; give others, especially those who I have the most trouble with, the love and respect I desire.

Summary

- Once you develop a comfortable system of recording your dreams, doing so will become habitual, freeing your attention for other things.
- Recording in 1st-person, present tense and giving your dream a title are both ways to help you to bring it back to life in the present moment.
- In choosing a dream to work with, initially err on the side of simplicity and brevity.
- Identifying life issues will allow you to compare your priorities to those of your interviewed characters, which will become clear as you interview them. Are they the same? If they are different, what does that imply?

Notes

1 If you know a creative genius who has the ability to create such a program and who is also interested in IDL, have him or her contact us via DreamYoga.com

2 In their emphasis on goodness and love, Western religious traditions create a repressed devil of evil, sin, and guilt. Hinduism and Buddhism, in their emphasis on transcendent truth and reality, repress *avidya,* which is both ignorance and illusion. While such an emphasis is a healthy antidote to the self-deprecation inherent in any notion of original sin, it creates irresolvable epistemological problems, dividing reality into relative and absolute truth, neither of which satisfy the other. IDL does not make this distinction because to do so creates a false dichotomy between truth and illusion that is not reflected in the

comments of many interviewed emerging potentials. It is false because our experience at this moment has whatever degree of reality or illusion that we bring to it. In addition to being a false distinction, it is unhelpful, in that it discounts experiences that we decide are unreal, illusory, or less real. It is also unhelpful because knowing what is real and what is true does not necessarily translate into right action. Consequently, IDL focuses not on issues of what is good or what is real but on clarifying your priorities. It assumes that health, balance, and transformation follow from the alignment of your waking identity with the priorities of life, as reflected by those of your life compass. These are revealed by the preferences of a cross-section of your interviewed emerging potentials. This is an operational definition of getting unstuck and one that is falsifiable.

3   The majority of priorities are not supposed to be transformative, because transformation is a relatively rare occurrence. Expect to spend some 80% of your time in *thesis*, when you focus on balancing your roles, learning new skills, and moving from unconscious incompetence to unconscious competence. Expect to spend perhaps 15% of your time in *antithesis*, or serious conflict, stress, distress, or turmoil. Antithesis is a requirement and pre-requisite for transformation. However, conflict and stress can be normal and healthy, as when we develop symptoms related to our bodies fighting off a virus, bacterial infection or other disease, exercise, or are challenged to learn new career skills. Part of what makes IDL effective is its ability to turn aversive *antithesis* into important, worthwhile, meaningful, and valued experiences. You will be fortunate if you spend 5% of your time in transformation; few do. However, it is a mistake to get impatient and attempt to force *synthesis*, as people do when they take hallucinogens, undergo excessive purifications, or are on visionquests. Such experiences can temporarily alter your state, like orgasm, but such experiences rarely translate into lasting stable transformation.

Chapter 7

Purpose of the Dream Sociomatrix

Those roles that you play out of your awareness play you. No one is completely free who is victimized by their unconscious identification with roles. Those roles that you do not own are externalized, first internally, then externally.

The importance of such roles is typically underestimated. Starke R. Hathaway, the creator of the MMPI, the Minnesota Multiphasic Personality Inventory, a standard and highly respected diagnostic tool long used in the mental health field, notes that such roles both define and create personality.

> A kind of lying or role playing (if you must use a euphemism) is inevitably a part of personality . . . It is obvious that we provide a physician, a bartender, an employer and a spouse with different views of ourselves. One cannot say which of you is the real person. The real person you speak of is usually a vaguely described confidential self that you see in yourself or others. But such confidential selves are roles too and much less useful ones for most purposes than are the routine ones of your daily encounters . . . I still feel, as I have for some time, that no subject is more important for your work with personality measurement than is role playing, or perhaps, better, multiple personality. We need to know the various personalities of an individual and the motivational factors influencing their appearance . . . interpretation of test data can proceed validly only when you can have an idea which personality the testee has presented.[1]

Dream Sociometry is a process by which you can take responsibility for roles you have unconsciously created, thereby withdrawing their unconscious externalization in ways that undercut health, relationships, and peace of mind. It also introduces you to new roles that have never been a part of your identity, as well as reframes roles that have been in transformative ways.

The Dream Sociomatrix and resulting commentaries support many of the goals of IDL. These include to

- provide a self-directed dreamwork methodology which supports the ends of IDL;
- provide a method by which waking events can be evaluated as if they were recalled dreams;

- collect, record and quantify preferences regarding your perspectives, thoughts, feelings, and actions;
- support healthy waking choices based on a broad-based internal consensus;
- provide objectivity for self-appraisal;
- offer a personally convincing exploration of a dream narrative;
- provide data by which a Dream Sociogram can be created, which itself serves as a research tool;
- support and encourage clarity, lucidity, waking up, and enlightenment through identification with transformational emerging potentials.

Purpose of the Dream Sociomatrix

- support the reduction of nightmares and dream drama;
- re-own multiple projected perspectives in order to stop externalizing your wake-up calls;
- indicate the degree and nature of internal conflict associated with your particular life issues;
- expand and thereby grow your sense of self out of fixations, woundings, and limitations;
- support consolidation, the stability of your functioning at your current level of development as a pre-requisite for transformation by identifying, listening to and addressing the needs of rejected, abandoned, or ignored perspectives which are vital to your growth;
- increase your ability to see all others as personified perspectives, thereby treating them as you would want to be treated;
- understand the life issues of concern to your interviewed characters;
- understand the priorities of life and your life compass and their relationship to your own;
- recognize the perspective of the intrasocial context as a whole, that is, of Dream Self, interviewed characters, and Dream Consciousness;
- indicate the amount of internal cohesiveness, integration, and synergism present within your intrasocial groups;
- develop an innate knowingness, spontaneity, and an increased capacity for intimacy;
- foster conflict resolution skills;
- provide a foundation for ongoing constructive life change, increasing wakefulness, lucidity, clarity, and enlightenment;
- support transformation, your evolution to your next highest level of development
- increase the likelihood that transformation lasts, when it does occur;
- support transpersonal development through disidentification with your waking identity while identifying with increasingly interdependent and transcendent perspectives;
- support the stable ability to witness yourself while awake, dreaming, and deeply asleep.

A method of self-disclosure through character identification

The best way of successfully acting a part is to be it.

Arthur Conan Doyle

The Dream Sociomatrix is designed to gather and group the preferences of the characters you have chosen to interview. Interviewing is done by "becoming" characters in the dream or life drama and asking them questions. When you become an interviewed character from a dream narrative, you merge with it and look out at your life from its perspective. Your identity is no longer primarily that of your waking self. You are, to the best of your ability, speaking as the identity of that particular interviewed character, regardless of what it is. While character identification implies empathy, it is more than empathy. Empathy involves imagining that you are taking the perspective of another as you consider their needs. Character identification is beyond this. It involves *identification* with the needs of the other while both sympathy and empathy imply a differentiation of identities. What differentiates character identification is the conscious and arbitrary nature of the identification in not only an emotional but a conceptual way.

Uses of the Dream Sociomatrix evaluation

Clarifying the structure of a intrasocial group clarifies *your* internal structure. Understanding the perspectives of individual members within intrasocial group discloses which emerging potentials you accept, reject, or ignore and for what reasons. Perhaps more importantly, you discover which emerging potentials accept, reject, or ignore *you* and why they do so. Evaluation of the Dream Sociomatrix identifies intrapersonal conflicts so that you may more clearly understand how you sabotage your own development. Such objectivity is invaluable. It also has a remarkable unassailability and intimacy that is often lacking in traditional sources of objectivity, such as psychotherapy. Evaluating the Dream Sociomatrix allows you to diagnose the interior relationships that impinge on the resolution of your various life issues. You will gain a sense of just what perspectives are invested in the perspectives that they hold and why.

However, the real power of collecting interviewed character preferences does not come from your evaluation of those preferences and how they relate to other preferences and your life behaviors. Becoming dream characters breaks down your rigid identification with role-based definitions of self. This allows personal self-definitions to slowly be replaced by transpersonal, life compass based self-definitions. This is absolutely essential if growth is going to continue beyond the mid-personal developmental levels. Such a process provides an experiential broadening of identity that is not based on a cognitive grasp of truth. While this objective can be accomplished in a number of ways, few are as accessible or as effective as successive identification with relatively objective perspectives.

In addition to providing all of these resources, the Dream Sociomatrix provides the source data to create the Dream Sociogram where previously obscure choices, motivational forces, and internal relationships are clarified. Important information about how you choose, when you choose, what you choose, and how you feel about the choices that you make becomes accessible, providing an opportunity for improved decision making. Interviewing characters also supports the expression of elaborations that clarify your life issues. These are noted in the Dream Sociomatrix Commentary, which is created in tandem with the Dream Sociomatrix.

Once preferences are stated numerically they can be tabulated, producing data that allows patterns of intrasocial interaction to be mapped in the Dream Sociogram. This allows you to take a bird's eye view of factors and relationships that create and maintain your identity. Essentially, it is a perspective that metaphorically transcends all form, including the identifications that create your thoughts, feelings, and perspectives, whether conscious or unconscious. To create the Dream Sociomatrix, dream elements are first listed, classified, and placed into one of the three categories described in the next chapter.

Summary

- By learning to complete Dream Sociomatrices students of IDL gain an in-depth experience of the principles underlying IDL character interviewing techniques.
- Because the transpersonal is an experiential dimension that includes the cognitive and belief-based world views, experiential methodologies such as Dream Sociometry are required to access it.
- Identification with characters listed in the Dream Sociomatrix can provide a powerful way to assimilate perspectives that echo priorities of your life compass into your waking consciousness.

Note

1 In the Foreword to the first (1960) edition of the MMPI Handbook. (1972). Dahlstorm, Welsh, & Dahstrom, pp. ix–x)

Bibliography

Dahlstorm, L., Welsh, G. S., & Dahstrom, L. E. (1972). *MMPI handbook*. Univ. of Minnesota Press

Chapter 8

The dream elements

Every man is a divinity in disguise, a god playing the fool.

Ralph Waldo Emerson

Dream elements fall into three broad categories: characters, actions, and feelings. IDL assumes that your dream elements manifest specific aspects not only of your identity, but of life itself. They amplify different truths about both you and who you can potentially become. Their interactional patterns indicate the context in which these truths manifest in your life. In addition, they reflect realities that transcend and include your identity. This is because they are not generated by *you*. They are as much a creation of the other characters in the dream or waking drama as they are yours. Therefore, when you grasp these broader patterns, you expand your sense of self. This is clearly seen by the meanings given to characters, feelings, and actions by the perspectives that you interview while creating a Dream Sociomatrix. This working hypothesis, that these three categories of elements both represent aspects of your identity and unborn yet emerging broader and potential definitions of who you are, has several advantages. First, it requires you to take responsibility for whatever you experience in your dream, since you are dealing with self-aspects. Second, it requires that you suspend your psychological geocentrism, or your assumption that the dream or life drama is all about *you*. Third, it opens you to spontaneity and creativity in your awakening and enlightenment that is simply impossible when growth is framed in terms of the limited context of your identity, however you care to define it. While you are encouraged to start creating a Dream Sociogram with these assumptions, remember that each interviewed perspective will, in its own time and way, provide you with its own opinion of what it is and is not.

Interviewed characters personify perspectives, actions, and feelings with which you identify, whether or not you are aware of them. "Dream character" or "interviewed perspective" refers to an interviewed identity *with* its associated actions, opinions, feelings, beliefs, ideals, and world view. Normally, you are in the process of becoming more and more locked into your thoughts, feelings, behaviors, and relationships through your repetitious and mostly unconscious preferences.

An interviewed character like a house is different from dream actions and feelings because it necessarily includes action states and feelings, even if these actions and feelings are "doing nothing" and "having no feelings." Interviewed characters model, exemplify, or manifest actions or feelings, while an action or feeling is not necessarily an expression of some particular identity. This is why it is easier to give voice to an interviewed character than it is to a dream action or feeling.

Dream actions and emotions indicate properties possessed by or describing interviewed characters and their interactions. Action elements express metaphorically what some role you take does, whether or not you are aware of it. They indicate various problem-solving strategies you are employing, your modes of conflict resolution, and your approaches to stress management. They are predictive of life issues you will confront in the future. Emotional elements express what some role that you take feels. If an interviewed character is angry, you are angry. If an interviewed character says that it is shameful and does not deserve to be alive, you are talking about yourself. Acknowledging and taking responsibility for all the feelings that exist in an intrasocial group is a difficult but necessary step toward greater honesty, courage, intuition, intimacy, and compassion. It is in this area that Dream Sociometry may perhaps provide the greatest opportunity for therapeutic catharsis as an aid to personal and transpersonal development.

Interviewed characters forms with emotions and behaviors

You are a collection of mirrors reflecting what everyone else expects of you. When we speak of your interviewed characters in the context of their intrasocial existence, together with the actions and feelings with which they are identified, they are *forms* or concrete *holons*. A "form" is an identity or "being." A "holon" is a part-whole that includes consciousness, feelings and thoughts in the interior individual quadrant, behaviors in the exterior individual quadrant, relationships in the exterior collective quadrant, and interpretations, values, and world views in the interior collective quadrant. Holons are concrete in that they are more solid, stable, and distinct than thoughts and feelings. Interviewed characters are forms that *have* thoughts and feelings. They are reflections of your preferences, which are themselves feelings, both acknowledged and disowned. Dream Sociometry assumes that interviewed characters are intrasocial roles and personifications of your feelings, actions, and thoughts.

Dream perspectives are personified as distinct and concrete *forms* within the context of an intrasocial group. An interviewed character is a "form" in that it specifies a relatively substantial and crystallized identity. This is why character

Dream Sociometric scores are placed on the form axis of the Dream Sociogram. They are the dream elements that most closely parallel the "matter" of your waking world. They are the dream equivalent of "substance," a manifestation of the adage, "thoughts are things." More fundamentally, interviewed characters are incarnations of your purposes and intentions, your outlook on life, your world view, your zeitgeist. These are interior collective holonic characteristics manifesting or expressing themselves in the exterior individual quadrant as specific *things*. Interviewed characters are therefore not fundamentally processes or emotions, although they possess action states of being (sitting, talking, listening, etc.) and express emotions every time they state preferences. Many interviewed characters also possess feelings (a happy child, an independent skunk, a peaceful tree). Interviewed characters are personifications of perspectives toward life that you typically do not consciously own but that nevertheless shape your perceptions and your options.

Beings, objects, and things convey attitudes you hold

Interviewed characters are not only "beings." They are objects and things, like rocks, keys, atoms, goblins, planets, deities, fungi, clouds, and fire. How is it that interviewed characters personify aspects of your identity? While you certainly identify with your feelings and your actions (we "get" mad, "feel" afraid, or "do" a deed,) you are even more likely to consider yourself to *be* your beliefs, your perspectives, and your thoughts. Your perspectives and thoughts are no more who you truly are than are your behaviors and feelings, even if you happen to be more closely identified with them. They often indicate the more engrained level of identification of your current proximate self, which you are destined to outgrow in time.

Actions can become interviewed dream characters

Interviewed characters are in fact action processes that constellate into a definite identity: hurricanes, cancer, fire, night, or a migraine headache. We simply are not used to thinking of some "things," such as people and objects as processes. For example, "foreign" viruses and bacteria by far outnumber human cells and are indeed necessary for our survival, but we do not think of ourselves as the intermingling and interaction of an amazing variety of life processes but as a *self* or *entity*. Groups of objects, which are themselves processes, are typically classified as one interviewed character (igneous rocks, cerebral dendrites, ocean waves, dandelions). One member of a homogeneous group may represent the entire group (gang leader, one bolt of lightning in a thunderstorm, parade member).

Interviewed dream characters are choosers

Because interviewed characters are the dream carriers of purpose and intention, they manifest as *choosers*. They often state in their elaborations in the various commentaries that they choose who and what they are and how they will act in a particular dream. Whether this is indeed the case or whether they are in fact predetermined by broader factors, such as Dream Consciousness, is probably a matter of perspective. The choices these characters make are stated as preferences within the Dream Sociomatrix. They can differ not only in valence and intensity, but also in degree of overtness. For example, in one dream about chickens, many choices are made, but by who and for what? Why chickens on a conveyor belt? Why not have sides of beef on meat hooks? Why does the conveyor belt choose to like the movement of chickens upon it, while the chickens do not? Why doesn't the conveyor belt hate the movement of chickens on it, while the chickens love it instead? What does it mean that most of the choices expressed in any dream narrative are merely implied and are largely unknown to us until we interview various perspectives, actors, forms, holons, or dream characters? What impact do their unrecognized preferences have on your health and your waking life? All of these questions can only be answered by asking the appropriate interviewed character to state and elaborate on their preferences because the questions themselves are not even revealed until these choosers are recognized.

Unknown to you, you constantly share both your power and control over your life with these choosers. If you align with them, great things happen. If you set yourself against them, which remains the prevailing stage of human evolution, unintended consequences happen.

Interviewed characters are chosen

Not only do you choose how you are going to view and treat your fellow interviewed characters, *they* are choosing how *they* are going to view, treat, and feel about *you*. For example, a dream monster or villain gets to choose whether to attack you or not. A dream tree gets to choose whether it stays planted or floats in the air. You may be preferred, rejected, or simply ignored by any interviewed character and each of these preferences not only do not belong to you; they have consequences. What are the consequences of their decisions regarding how to relate to you? Do they create integration or disintegration, unity or conflict? When you are dreaming, or when you are lost in the life drama that is the topic of your Dream Sociomatrix, how objective and aware are your choices toward its various component forms, holons, entities, substances, identities or characters? Are your choices based on ignorance, fear, and illusion or on wisdom, respect, and truth? If you are unaware of the patterns of preferences of other dream characters, how can you accurately perceive their intentions? If your choices, whether dreaming or awake, are based on ignorance, fear, and illusion, then will you not often choose unhealthy or simply unproductive relationships with them?

From egocentrism to polycentrism

When dream characters are considered to be perspectives rather than symbols, an entirely different category of questions is raised, not only about the dream, but also about yourself. Instead of asking, "*What does this character represent in my life?*" You ask, "*As this interviewed perspective, who and what am I choosing to be?*" Instead of asking, "*How does this dream fit into my psychological world and relate to my waking life?*" You are asking, "*How do I, as Dream Self, fit into this intrasocial world?*" "*How do my needs relate to the priorities of this group?*" When you ask these questions, your relationship with your microcosm becomes drastically altered. Your waking identity is no longer the center of your universe; you move from a psychological egocentrism or geocentrism to a polycentrism and multiperspectivalism which has at least as much reality and relevance as does your role-based, social universe.

Interviewed characters are created by patterns of attitude

Where do your interviewed characters come from? While there are other possible, highly significant non-waking sources of interviewed characters, such as subconscious complexes, past life identities, totem animals, different dimensions, and disincarnates, your waking reality is by far the largest and most parsimonious source of dream issues and interviewed characters. While your dream characters *could* be created by God or dolphins from the Pleiades, or be thought implants by the machines that generate the "matrix," a far simpler and therefore more likely explanation is that you created them but didn't realize it. Thinking involves an internal, sub-vocal dialogue among differing perspectives and preferences concerning your perspectives, behaviors, and feelings. Thought exemplifies your various perceptual frameworks and roles. When these waking attitudinal patterns and social and psychological roles are personified as perspectives or patterns in your dreams, they manifest as interviewed characters.

The problem is that those who arrive at this conclusion settle on one reductionistic possibility that closes off other aspects of the human holon. Reality is self-created, not collectively created. Reality is individually generated, not externally supplied. However, reality refuses to be reduced to one or another of the four quadrants of any holon and to do so not only abuses it; it disempowers us by cutting us off from profound sources of creativity and transformation.

Interviewed characters may be usefully considered to be components of underlying, synthesizing norms or patterns which IDL generally refers to as "perspectives." This term is itself a nod to the generative nature of the internal collective quadrant of the human holon. As your feelings and needs form

the core of your waking perspectives and beliefs, so inner values and purposes crystallize into interviewed characters. For instance, in *Disfigured Woman*,
feelings of ugliness, fear, and unacceptability create a very definite and powerful interviewed character, the disfigured woman. In *Methodical Suicide*, self-
condemnation manifests as *hari-kari* by the Man who embodies self-hatred by
killing himself.

Because intrasocial groups, that is, collections of interviewed perspectives,
whether from dreams or waking life, provide so much valuable information on
the formation and alteration of perspectives, it is a pity that social psychologists
and sociologists have not paid more attention to them. Because interviewed
characters embody thoughts, beliefs and purposes, as well as perspectives, the
terms "perspective" and "world view" often seem more appropriate than "perspective" to describe them. In any case, these are all internal collective, herme-
neutic realities that create liberating contexts.

Interviewed dream character roles are generally mundane and repetitive

Because you have countless perspectives and perspectives you have an endless
variety of interviewed characters that populate your dreams. Most of us, however, have highly predictable patterns of interviewed character interaction due
to our cultural and environmental commonalties. Research into dream content
analysis has shown this to be the case. Just as there exist relatively few basic
emotions and colors of the spectrum, so are there a limited number of thematic
patterns with which intrasocial groups normally concern themselves. Themes
generally cluster around emotions. For example, themes of abandonment, attack,
and avoidance are based on fear. Themes of loneliness, hopelessness, helpless-
ness, and powerlessness are based on sadness and depression. Themes of forgetfulness are based on confusion. Themes of aggression and abuse are based on
anger. One can also look at these in terms of an even simpler model: all themes
will relate to either persecutor, victim, or rescuer roles in the Drama Triangle
or else represent a theme of disengagement from it. You may have many different interviewed characters, but they generally depict a handful of repetitive
themes or life issues. While different intrasocial groups, that is, constellations of
interviewed perspectives, will give you insight into these life issues, the issues
themselves tend to be relatively stable. While it does not take work on many
dreams and life dramas in order to identify your core issues and greatly impact
the damage created by chronic dysfunctional life patterns, it takes regular application of IDL to stabilize and maintain a higher level of development.

It has long been recognized that specific personalities convey discrete and
specific perspectives or approaches to dealing with life. Daniel Boone conjures
up a pioneering life for Americans. The four-headed Roman deity Janus is
often seen as a metaphor for omniscience. A ghost might be associated with
fear or with openness to other states of awareness. For a Christian, a dream of

a dove or a fish might carry important religious significance. Depictions of the devil are effective ways of awakening themes of evil, death, sin and guilt. Such formulations are symbolic and archetypal, representing widely held perspectives or perspectives. It is in this sense that interviewed characters are crystallized, materialized points of view that you hold. Your purpose here, however, is not to explore interviewed characters from the conceptual framework of symbol or archetype. This has been done magnificently elsewhere.[1] Dream Sociometry does not ask, "What is the archetypal significance of this interviewed character?" Instead, it asks, "Who do I, as this interviewed character, think that I am?" "How do I perceive my position and purpose in this group as this interviewed character?" "How do I relate to my fellow interviewed characters?" "What do I think of Dream Self?" "What do I think of waking identity and its choices?" Dream Sociometry does not ask, "What does this symbol or archetype tell me about my degree of individuation?" Instead, it asks, "What do I, as this interviewed character, have to say about the intrasocial reality of which this waking individual is but one component?"

Taking the phenomenological perspective

Menard Boss has noted that

> in your dreams you experience real physical facts: a thing is a real thing, an animal is a real animal, a man is a real man and a ghost is a real ghost. In your dreams you are in just as real a material world as in your waking life.[2]

It is hardly enough to say that your interviewed characters are crystallized, materialized points of view that you hold; they indicate much more. Your interviewed characters are not simply visual metaphors for waking perspectives. They do not consider *themselves* to be symbolic; why should you consider them to be so? Your interviewed characters are, at the very least, who and what they say that they are. They represent *themselves*. In the universe in which they operate, interviewed characters are not only *real*, they are as real within their cognitive framework as you are in yours. They are as real as is any other consensus reality. To discover the nature of their world view you must move into that dimension through a willingness to see that world from their perspective. When you do so, you suspend your assumptions about reality and illusion and approach the dream narrative or life drama from a thoroughgoing phenomenological perspective. Dream interpretation is best provided by *them* and in the context of your respect for the self-transcending sociocultural matrix to which they belong.

The life situations depicted by intrasocial depictions of dreams and life dramas cannot be equated with or reduced to waking reality because our waking perspective is singular and that provided by Dream Sociometry is multi-perspectival. Although we take many waking roles, as noted above, these are generally experienced in a temporally linear fashion by one perspective – our waking identity. The source and explanation for intrasocial reality are therefore not found in a relating of events back to waking reality. Still, that approach is generally the only alternative most people recognize, because they habitually approach dreamwork out of their waking context.

You find yourself in a position similar to a catfish within its own watery universe trying to perceive a tree or a bird on the bank. How can it see life otherwise than it does? Humans, however, have other possibilities of perception, available through meditation, lucid dreaming, and empathy. Other universes are open to you that are not open to a fish, but only if you are willing to let go of those biases inherent in any waking perspective. As you do so, you can begin to understand that interviewed characters express a great deal more about you than is available if you only look at life through your waking perspective. Some interviewed characters that you will meet will amaze you with the clarity of their purpose, knowingness, acceptance and compassion.

Crystallization of feelings, actions, and attitudes

Interviewed characters also embody the crystallization or precipitation of life frequencies personified as forms. Intentions and feelings are interviewed characters in the making. Interviewed characters contain elements of affect (or energy) and action (or process) in addition to perspective or perspective. A dream dragon, for instance, may convey feelings of fear, although the dragon is asleep, and angry actions, although he is munching daisies. While emotions express *how* the interviewed character chooses to be and actions express *what* the interviewed character chooses to be, interviewed characters define *who* the individual chooses to be in the particular life situations metaphorically depicted by the dream narrative or life drama. In Dream Sociometry, you imaginatively identify with interviewed characters and not dream feelings and actions, but only because it is easier to imagine oneself a "who" than a "what" or a "how."

Interviewing dream characters provides transformational perspectives

Your Dream Self is a special kind of interviewed character who generally serves as a surrogate for your waking perspectives toward this or that life issue. Let us say you remember a dream of losing your keys. The dream seems pretty straightforward. You think, "My disorganization and forgetfulness is getting to me." However, the life issue often transcends the straightforward concerns of your waking identity. Therefore, other interviewed characters confront Dream Self with other perspectives on the issue. When you interview the keys, they may something like, "We're not lost. We know exactly where we are. You need to chill." This response invites the dreamer to see the problem not as her disorganization and forgetfulness but as her anxiety and self-criticism *about* her disorganization and forgetfulness! This may seem like a subtle shift, but it is fundamental and powerful. Dream Self often merely reflects your waking orientation toward your life issues. That is why much dream interpretation only ends up validating waking perspectives. You run from a monster, you run from responsibilities; you fall off cliffs, you lose control over your eating, drinking, or sexual habits. For the monster, however, the issue is rarely avoidance of responsibilities; it may be anger at being ignored. For the cliff, the issue is rarely loss of control; instead, it may involve respect for natural limits. If you fail to take these perspectives into account, you stay stuck in conflict, ignorant of yourself.

Just as Dream Self is only one aspect of a intrasocial group, so your waking perception of who you are is only one portion of the totality of your waking experience. Your waking experience is itself only a small portion of the totality of those perspectives that are available to you. For the most part, you naively assume that you are awake while you are taking part in a dream. As you shall see, the placement of your Dream Self in the Dream Sociogram reflects your degree of awareness of and concern about the life issues expressed by the intrasocial group.

About modifiers

Interviewed characters are often accompanied by modifiers: a *blue* Mercedes, a *short* chimpanzee, an *ugly* matron. Normally these modifiers are considered in Dream Sociometry to be aspects of the interviewed character and are not listed separately as they would be in say, dream content analysis. Some modifiers, however, refer to actions or feelings, as in a *drunk* chimpanzee or a *jovial* gerbil. Such modifiers are considered to be separate elements and can be noted in the Dream Sociomatrix as such.

Dream Consciousness: an extraordinary perspective

You have the option to also interview Dream Consciousness, the perspective that represents the womb out of which the dream or life drama flows. To do so, place it at the end of your list of *choosing* interviewed characters, at the bottom of the left-hand column of choosing interviewed characters. You may also place it as a *chosen* dream element at the end of the chronological listing of dream elements along the top border of the Dream Sociomatrix.

There are several reasons why you might want to take this rather advanced step, one that is not included in any of the examples provided in this text. Identification with Dream Consciousness provides practice experiencing the dream and therefore your life, from the perspective that transcends form. As such, it is a metaphor for causal witnessing. Experiencing yourself as formless witness strengthens that experience in your awareness, improving your access to it in meditation and at other times. In addition, identification with Dream Consciousness provides opportunities to experience the eighth and most rarified of preferences: choosing to take a perspective that transcends all preferences. This is a very subtle and sophisticated stance, rarely noted in Dream Sociomatrices, and if any dream voice is most likely to consistently provide opportunities to grow into it, Dream Consciousness would be that voice.

Although Dream Consciousness is not a dream of life drama character, interview Dream Consciousness just as you would any interviewed character. It will probably express preferences. Note any elaborations in the Dream Sociomatrix Commentary, just as you would for any interviewed character.[3]

Actions

Actions are dream elements describing dream processes and interactions

Actions are those dream elements that indicate processes of interviewed characters and relationships among elements. They describe interactions, the quality and quantity of the energy flow within a dream pattern, and often the life issues that the intrasocial group personifies. Action is the category of dream element that most closely approximates the behavioral aspect of your waking world, including the activities of thought, overt and covert behaviors, interactions among people, and the manipulation of objects. They are generally recorded as verbs in the dream narrative. Any dream element that is primarily a process is considered to be an action.

Examples of dream actions

Being out of breath describes a behavior and is listed as an action as does "not bleeding." Thinking, seeing, astral projection, listening to your deceased grandfather, doing nothing, changing into another interviewed character, being creative, climbing, meditating, sleeping, swimming, having an intuition, gawking, and dying are all dream actions. Potential actions such as "strength," "will," or "chastity" are also included in this category. Actions also define the direction of flow of the life force that animates the dream. Times, such as the 19th century, 3:35 P.M., or daybreak, are processes and categorized as actions.

Action modifiers

As mentioned above, interviewed characters are often described or modified by words such as cruelty, shyness, cleverness, etc. These traits are categorized as *actions*. Sometimes interviewed characters are described in terms of role performance or the action expressed: teacher, racecar driver, yodeler, rapids, or thunderstorm. These elements will usually be classified as interviewed characters, not actions.

Emotions

The varieties of dream emotion

Albert Einstein noted that

> *Everything that the human race has done and thought is concerned with the satisfaction of deeply felt needs and the assuagement of pain. One has to keep this constantly in mind if one wishes to understand transpersonal movements and their development. Feeling and desire are the motive forces behind all human endeavor and human creation, in however exalted a guise the latter may present itself to us.*[4]

We have said that your interviewed characters are reflections of your preferences. Preferences are most fundamentally feelings. In a sense, interviewed characters are precipitates of your preferences and feelings. Dream emotions indicate your different affective states: sadness, happiness, fear, disgust, anger, confusion, joy, equanimity, boredom, spontaneity, and impatience. Some examples of feelings taken from dream narratives include: pleased, surprised, dedication, excited, wanting to go, (eagerness), fun (happy), curious, awkward, and relieved.

As you can see from some of these examples, dream feelings come in many varieties. There are infinite hues of emotional expression, just as there are endless shades of color in the spectrum. Just as there are primary colors that create a multitude of shades when combined, so there are primary emotions from which all other emotions are derived. Examples of primary emotions are pleasure, anxiety, irritation, sadness, confusion, and excitement.[5]

A feeling is an intensity

An emotion is not a "thing" in the sense that an object or even a thought is. A feeling is an intensity, a quality, the electricity that runs through the wires – not the wires themselves, nor the act of "running." Emotions communicate purpose by their type, quantity and use. In *A Robber Is Killed*, the Burglar is scared because he is caught in the act. In *Seeking Privacy*, Dream Self wants privacy for sex he feels conflicted about. Any dream element that is relatively formless and energized is considered an emotion.

The most basic level of dream expression

Many contemporary psychologists consider emotional expression to be a type of behavior, a form of mental action. Such an approach, although reductionistic, is valuable in that it emphasizes the accessibility of inner states to behavioral modification. As you shall see, emotions often anchor dream experiences more clearly to waking patterns than do dream actions and interviewed characters. Recognizing and identifying dream emotions and patterns of affect is the first and most important tool for relating a dream to waking life issues. But feelings are more than behaviors, traits, or characteristics. On the contrary, dream feelings often seem to precipitate into the individual dream identities we call interviewed characters. This is exactly opposite of waking life, in which *individuals* manifest feelings.

While emotions are the least common of the three categories of dream elements classified in Dream Sociometry, they are fundamental. Inchoate and often overlooked, they represent life force in a seminal, relatively unmanifest state when it is both undefined and potent. This relative lack of emotional elements in comparison to interviewed characters and actions may be due to nothing more than a habitual lack of awareness combined with a chronic lack of empathy for the feelings of other interviewed characters. Feelings enliven thoughts. Thoughts, actions, and personality are the clothes feelings wear. However, in Dream Sociometry, dream thoughts are not classified as feelings. Thinking, "Where did I put that shovel?" "Listening," or "saying to myself," are actions and are summarized and listed as such in the Dream Sociomatrix. Mental states with sub-vocal, auditory, or visual content are classified as actions. Dream emotions are often distilled into the crystallized form of some interviewed character, with actions defining the nature of the flow of the creative process from feeling into its personification as interviewed character. For instance, a witch casting a spell might be a crystallization of manipulative anger and a desire for revenge on others, or she could be a condensation of higher caring manifesting itself in a concrete way. The point is to understand how feelings are personified as interviewed characters, not to speculate or interpret what the witch "means." In Dream Sociometry, the witch will usually tell you what she is, why she is that way, what she wants, and how she relates to your life.

Negative and positive dream emotions

Because there are fewer basic emotions than there are actions or interviewed characters, learning to recognize dream feeling is a powerful tool for understanding patterns of life force. It is not unusual for humans to be aware of many more negative feelings than positive ones. While this may be due to our cultural grammatical preferences, it is certainly a sad commentary on man's current level of development. As you evolve in awareness, you will become aware of many more varieties of subtle pleasurable affective states. Meditative traditions are very clear in stating that there are many other positive states of awareness ahead of you on the spectrum of your personal evolution. Your dreams monitor and comment upon your emotional development as you work with applying specific dream feedback in your daily life.

Watch for hidden emotions

The Dream Sociomatrix Commentary tends to reveal emotions embedded in the personalities of various interviewed characters. A monster, for instance, can personify feelings of disgust at one's own ugly habits. Feelings often masquerade as actions, modifiers, or interviewed characters and may never be identified. You know this has occurred when, in the course of your interviewing, you come across an action or modifier in a dream narrative but sense that it is actually a feeling in disguise. Examples could include "generosity" (appreciation or kindness), "praise" (thankfulness), "*Am I inconsiderate?*" (self-doubt), "beautiful" (enjoyment), "complementary" (appreciative), "having enough" (satisfied), or "cut off" (lonely). Be aware of this common confusion, and learn to look for the feelings hidden in your dream actions. It is not unusual to find only one or two emotions named in a dream narrative but many more evoked by the act of stating preferences (which are degrees of like and dislike and therefore emotions) and expressed in commentary elaborations. This demonstrates how cut off we normally are from the depth and breadth of emotions that bring vitality to life.

Summary

- As choosers and chosen, your interviewed characters create your reality. You are both the subject and object of your experience, a victim only when you fail to listen to emerging potentials.
- Every preference is a choice, and every choice is an action. The identification and clarification of your actions and their consequences create the clarity you need to make better choices.
- While every preference is a feeling, interviewed characters also embody feeling states. These are relatively overt statements of the part affect plays in the expression of life issues both in your dreams and in your waking life.

Notes

1 Stevens, A. (1982). *Archetypes A Natural History of the Self*. Quill, or Eliade, M. (1958). *Patterns in Comparative Religion*. New York: World Pub. Co.
2 Boss, Medard, M. D. (1974). *The Analysis of Dreams*. In R. L. Wood & H. B. Greenhouse (Eds.), *The New World of Dreams* (p. 226). New York: Palgrave MacMillan.
3 Could you have a dream in which Dream Consciousness is an interviewed character? Yes, but then you have to ask the question, "What shall we call the perspective that dreamed a dream in which Dream Consciousness is a character? The name "Dream Consciousness" is a place holder for that perspective rather than an entity. Compare this with the concept of God, who is more than a place holder; God is a supreme *being*. Therefore, as a reality with substance, God can conceivably be a character in your dream. In fact many people, including Carl Jung, have had dreams in which God was a character. Dream Consciousness is formless. It transcends, by definition, any character, because it is that consciousness that generates or creates all conceivable forms. In *Dream Sociometry*, Dream Consciousness

can be both interviewer and interviewed, not as a dream character, but as the context which generated the dream.

4   Religion and Science. *New York Times Magazine*, November 9, 1930, pp. 1–4.

5   These are not primary feelings in the sense that they are most fundamental; Wilber gives the evolution of affect as beginning with reactivity, sensations, and physiostates such as touch, temperature, pleasure, and pain. Out of these evolve the "protoemotions" of tension, fear, rage and satisfaction, followed by the second-degree emotions of anxiety, anger, wishing, liking, and safety. Next come the third-degree emotions of love, joy, depression, hate, and belongingness. Fourth-degree emotions include universal affect, global justice, care, compassion, all-human love, and world-centric altruism. Beyond these are transpersonal affective states, including psychic level awe, rapture, all-species love, and compassion; subtle level ananda, ecstasy love-bliss, and saintly commitment; and causal-level infinite freedom-release and bodhisattvic-compassion followed by a transcendence of all affect in the non-dual state Wilber calls "One Taste." Wilber has correlated the evolution of the affective developmental line with basic developmental structures and many other factors on p. 198 of *Integral Psychology* (2000). Boston: Shambhala.

Bibliography

Boss, Medard, M. D. (1974). The analysis of dreams. In R. L. Wood & H. B. Greenhouse (Eds.), *The new world of dreams* (p. 226). New York: Palgrave MacMillan.

Eliade, M. (1958). *Patterns in comparative religion.* New York: World Pub. Co.

Stevens, A. (1982). *Archetypes: A natural history of the self.* Fort Mill, SC: Quill.

Chapter 9

Element categorization

Each interviewed character is a microcosm. Its physical body is the form through which the macrocosm manifests in your dream or life drama. Its mental/emotional nature is comprised of those thoughts, perspectives, and feelings that it expresses in the dream and in the dream commentaries. Its transpersonal nature is expressed by the life force that it embodies. Each interviewed character is non-dual life masked by form. Follow any interviewed character back to its source and you will experience awakening, clarity, lucidity, and enlightenment.

Determining categories

You will be deciding in which category to place some or all of your recalled dream elements. At times, you will have to make an arbitrary decision about which category an element belongs in. Element classification in Dream Sociometry is both less precise and less important than it is in dream content analysis. Your purpose is to teach yourself to deeply listen to a wide array of perspectives and then to demonstrate to them your respect by applying some portion of that wisdom in a conscientious way in your daily life. Your purpose is also to transform your consciousness by disidentifying with your stuck waking identity and merging with other perspectives that are more developed or knowledgeable than you are. Consequently, precise element classification is not crucial to the success of your experience with Dream Sociometry. Learn the principles, but don't get too obsessive about them or you just might have dreams with interviewed characters scolding you and telling you to BACK OFF!

When in doubt, become the element

It is possible for emotions and actions to state preferences. For example, a fire is an action or process but is localized and often focuses as an entity that threatens or warms. The fact that emotions and actions are generally not used as character in in Dream Sociometry is simply a consequence of the relative difficulty in identifying with an action or a feeling. In addition, actions and feelings often belong to an actor. For instance, a "happy jumper" implies not only an emotion, "happy," and an actor, "jumper," but the act of jumping. However, "happy" and "jumping" are modifiers that clearly belong to an actor. In other instances, the distinction is less clear. It is not obvious what the process "burning" belongs to other than "fire," which is also a process. The implication is that fire is best treated as a choosing character. Experiment. You may have your dream actions and feelings express preferences if you wish.

When in doubt about how to classify a dream element, imagine that you *are* that element. Become the element. How do you feel toward some of the other dream elements? If you have no preferences, or have considerable difficulty getting into role although you have the demonstrated ability to do so, the element is probably not an interviewed character. Try classifying it as an action. From time to time, however, you will run upon a dream element which is definitely an interviewed character but which has no preferences, and you can learn a lot from this preferential neutrality.

Sometimes, you will just not know how to classify an element. In such cases, you can leave it out, or you can make the element an interviewed character and see what, if anything, it has to say. Doing so allows you to take responsibility for that perspective and to use it as a wake-up call. Let it explain itself to you.

Guidelines for categorization

1)   Identify the essence of a phrase. For instance, "*She looked as if she was about to scream*," describes an emotion (anger or fear, for instance,) not an action (screaming).
2)   Subordinate modifiers. Use the word "house" to stand for "big brown house." This is done as a form of shorthand to make listing in the Dream Sociomatrix easier.
3)   Become those elements that you cannot categorize. If the element has no preferences or feelings when you identify with it, consider it to be an action.
4)   If you still feel that the element is not an action, consider it to be an interviewed or chosen character.

All elements do not have to be listed

Element classification in Dream Sociometry is an individual and subjective process. It is not essential that you list every element or that you list each one in its proper category. It is important to list those you do include in chronological order. Because your purpose is not primarily to analyze dream structure, accuracy, and inclusiveness are not as important as applying this process to those elements you do list. Therefore, avoid obsessiveness or even worries about accuracy. Generally speaking, if you provide a broadly effective context, you will hear important wake-up calls and receive useful recommendations, both of which will propel you forward in your development. You may find it sufficient to work with only a portion of the elements in any particular dream or with only one segment. Unless you are doing research, it is much more important to understand preferences that create your life issues and determine your happiness than it is to do an exhaustive investigation of a particular dream. Naturally, your ability to categorize and list dream elements will improve as you gain experience with the method. You will find that you will learn which category best fits each particular dream element.

Summary

- You will get an enormous amount of helpful information from this process whether or not you always classify your dream elements appropriately, so don't worry about it. However, if you become addicted, the above guidelines should help.

Chapter 10

Making predictions

You can make predictions about what preferences will show up as you interview various characters. This process, along with stating your associations to your dream, nightmare or waking drama, serves as a pre-test that allows you to assess how well you know yourself. It is very easy to assume that you – your waking identity – created the various preferences that are expressed in the Dream Sociomatrix. If that is so, then you should be able to predict your preferences. If you created these preferences and you know your own mind, then you know which choosing character is most accepting of itself and its fellows, correct? You will also be able to successfully predict which character is least accepting or most rejecting of the group as well as which characters, actions, and feelings are most preferred and most rejected by the group.

Here are the categories of predictive questions:

Which character is most accepting of itself?
Which character is least accepting of itself?
Which character is most accepting of the group as a whole?
Which character is least accepting of the group as a whole?
Which character is most preferred by the group?
Which character is most rejected by the group?
Which action is most preferred by the group?
Which action is most rejected by the group?
Which feeling is most preferred by the group?
Which feeling is most rejected by the group?

After you complete your Dream Sociomatrix, you can check your answers. How did you do? How well were you able to predict implies how well you know your own mind, does it not?

What is implied, apart from a greater certainty that you do not know your own mind as well as you assume that you do, if you are not able to predict these preferences? By definition, a part or member of a group, cannot grasp the whole of which it is only one component. This is because it is subjectively embedded in a larger, broader context. The only way that it can do so is to suspend its own identity and become that broader context. When it does so, then it can indeed grasp the whole of which it is normally only one component. IDL assumes that your waking identity is only one component of your greater intrasocial identity. It tests this theory with experiments such as this pre-post test. It does not assume that this greater intrasocial identity is some static, all-encompassing self or identity, but rather a broader context or holon that lies within still broader contexts or holons. Patterns of group preference represent a broader context than your own because they are a combination of the perspectives of *all* polled emerging potentials, not just those of your waking identity. The result is that you will probably find that while you are accurate in some of your predictions that you are inaccurate in others.

There are exceptions to this rule. The smaller the intrasocial group is, such as the one in the following example, the more likely you are to predict preferences accurately. The less conflict that there is in a group, the more likely you are to predict preferences accurately. The more successful you are at neutralizing interfering intrasocial conflict the more likely your waking identity is to be in alignment with the priorities of your life compass. You should be able to predict those priorities more accurately and to act confidently on behalf of your greater intrasocial community. However, if you find you are not very good at these predictions and you also note that there are considerable negative preferences, your confidence in your ability to act in a way that reflects the will of your greater intrasocial community is ill-founded.

Predictions for *Ken Wilber Dies* are:

Most Accepting	Ken
Least Accepting:	Dream Self
Most Preferred Character:	Ken
Least Preferred Character:	Other Driver
Most Preferred Action:	none
Least Preferred Action:	killed
Most Preferred Emotion:	none
Least Preferred Emotion:	very upset

Emotions are generally easy to predict because there are relatively few of them in most intrasocial groups. Least accepting and least preferred elements may be rejecting and rejected, but not necessarily. This distinction is based on whether scores are merely the least positive or whether they are actually negative in total. There is always a least positive element if there is more than one of its kind, but there are not always elements with negative totals. Evaluating your predictions is covered in Chapter 29.

Chapter 11

Structure of the Dream Sociomatrix

One must know oneself. If this does not serve to discover truth, it at least serves as a rule of life and there is nothing better.

Blaise Pascal

The Dream Sociomatrix clarifies life issues

The information that you acquire from the Dream Sociomatrix regarding the interactional patterns of dream elements is valuable to your understanding of whatever life issues that express themselves in your dreams. For instance, in *Confidence Snow Skiing*, the dreamer gets confirmation that he is succeeding in overcoming doubt and fear regarding his work. In *Spider in the Car*, the dreamer gains understanding into how he enjoys scaring himself. In *Rob's Flaky Metamorphosis*, the dreamer faces how he sacrifices his integrity and considers ways to change.

Like other aspects of IDL, do not accept the hypothesis that your dreams express your life issues as an article of faith. That is both unnecessary and unwise. Instead follow the injunctions listed here; write down three current life issues as questions, and then ask several interviewed characters of your choice their opinion about them. Then, you can come to your own conclusions about whether your dreams provide relevant and insightful information about your current life issues.

The Dream Sociomatrix grid

The Dream Sociomatrix is basically a grid that is drawn on graph paper or a computer template. They can also be scrawled on scraps of paper, as I have done, from time to time, meaning that they can be pursued in monasteries, prisons, and on deserted islands. This grid-based structure is used to obtain interviewed character preferences, to tabulate them, and to then provide numerical data (in the case of the Dream Sociogram) and elaborative data with which to construct the Dream Commentaries, the Dream Sociogram and the Action Plan. In the

Table 11.1

Dream Sociomatrix

Author: Dillard
Dream Date: 8/27/01
Dream Name:
Ken Wilber Dies
Smx Date: 8/27/01

Choosers: / Chosen elements:	Dream Self	Ken Wilber	Girlfriend	Car	Second Car	- Head on Crash	- Killed	*Very Upset	Other Driver	Character Raw Scores	Acceptance Axis Totals	Character Ambivalence
Dream Self	2	3	1			/3	/3	/3	/2	6/11	/5	M
Ken Wilber	3	3	3	1		/3	/3	2	/2	12/8	4	M
Girlfriend	2	3	2	1	/2	/3	/3	2	/2	10/10	0	D
Car	2	2	2	2/1	/3	/3	/2	2	/3	10/12	/2	H
Second Car						/3	/3	2	/2	2/8	/6	L
Other Driver				1	/3	/3	3	/3		4/9	/5	M
Dream Consciousness	3	3	3					3	3	12	12	
El. Raw Scores	12	14	11	4/1	1/5	/18	/17	1/3	3/11			
El. Axis Totals	12	14	11	3	1/4	/18	/17	8	/8			
EL Ambivalence												

Scoring Key:

1 = like, 2 = like a lot, 3 = love;
/1 = dislike, /2 = dislike a lot, /3 = hate

blank = indifference
* = complete acceptance

"*" = feeling elements
"-" = action elements

figure below, the Dream Sociomatrix for the dream *Ken Wilber Dies*, you see an example of such a grid recording the likes and dislikes of interviewed characters toward each listed element (interviewed character, action, or emotion) in the dream.

Noting the elements in the Dream Sociomatrix

Character, action, and emotional elements in the dream or life drama are written along the top margin of the grid in order of appearance in the dream narrative. They can be given an alphabetical designation, as they are in this example, but it is not necessary. Actions are preceded by dashes, emotions by an asterisk. These are arbitrary designations used simply to differentiate among the three element types when plotting the scores on the three element axes of the Dream Sociogram. Interviewed characters are not preceded by any mark.

If you have not underlined the characters in your dream narrative, do so now. This makes it less likely you will overlook one in this next step. Down the left margin of the grid list no more than four of your underlined interviewed characters in the order of their appearance in the dream, always beginning with yourself as you appear in the dream, called "Dream Self."

Now, for your first Dream Sociomatrix, list no more than eight dream elements (interviewed characters, actions, and feelings) in their order of appearance (chronologically) along the top margin of the Dream Sociomatrix. The flow of time in the dream is represented by the progress of preferences from left to right in the Dream Sociomatrix. When listing dream elements for the Dream Sociomatrix, beware of the tendency to write each element in its grammatical order, which may not coincide with its actual temporal placement in the dream.

The act of defining and listing dream elements often clarifies meanings otherwise obscured by grammar. For instance, in *The Professor Is Leaving*, the written phrase "I think that I had better not depend on him too much" becomes one emotional element, "caution." Consequently, through defining and specifying elements to note in the Dream Sociomatrix, you enhance your awareness of what you experienced in the dream.

If a dream element is not noted in the dream narrative, but you later realize it is present in the dream, you may include it in the Dream Sociomatrix in parentheses (see 2/27/82: *Employer*). If you realize you have left out an important element after completing the Dream Sociomatrix, you can squeeze it in by writing its name at the top where it best fits in the flow of the dream narrative and then dividing the column below it to add its preferences.

Seven degrees of preference

Eight symbols, 3, /2, /1 and 1, 2, 3, and empty grid box establish the relative strength of the preferences interviewed characters hold toward all intrasocial group elements. Because minus signs are difficult to read in the Dream

Sociomatrix, particularly when there are ambivalent preferences (3/2, 1/1), slash marks are used to designate negative preferences. You may choose to use minus signs if you prefer.

/3 indicates that the element is overwhelmingly disliked (hated), value −3;
/2 indicates that the element is strongly disliked, value −2;
/1 indicates that the element is disliked, value −1;
3 indicates that the element is overwhelmingly liked (loved), value +3;
2 indicates that the element is strongly liked, value +2;
1 indicates that the element is liked, value +1;

A blank box indicates that the element is neither liked nor disliked and the chooser doesn't care or is indifferent, value 0.

On rare instances, most often seen in some scorings by Dream Consciousness, there exists acceptance that transcends yet includes love and hate. Such a score cannot be given a numerical designation and therefore cannot be noted numerically in the Dream Sociomatrix or be reflected in the placement of an element in the Dream Sociogram. However, some non-numerical designation, such as a dot, can be used to indicate that the chooser cares in a way that transcends all preferences.

When an interviewed character has a negative opinion toward himself or herself, the preference may be circled to call attention to it. This helps you to remember that an unusually negative self-rating exists. Self-loathing by an interviewed character is particularly significant as an indicator of particularly intense internal conflict.

All of these preferences are spontaneously expressed as you identify with and respond in turn as each choosing interviewed character, noted at the left margin, to each chosen dream element, noted above the Dream Sociomatrix. You begin with yourself in the dream or life drama, Dream Self and ask yourself, "How do I feel toward myself in this dream/life drama?" "Do I like, like a lot, love, dislike, dislike a lot, hate or not care about myself?" It is not unusual to feel ambivalence. Perhaps you hate yourself at one point in the dream and like yourself at another. You would give yourself a score of 1/3. Before you go on, take a moment to explain your preference in writing. Why do you feel the way you do toward yourself in this dream/life drama? You then proceed by asking the same questions toward the second element across the top of the Dream Sociomatrix and place your preference toward it in the box below its name that intersects with "Dream Self" in the Dream Sociogram. Again, write your explanation of your preferences as "elaborations" before proceeding to write your preferences toward the third element along the top. These written elaborations are collected under the heading "Dream Sociomatrix Commentary. Stating your preferences, first as yourself and then as several other characters in the dream and, finally, as Dream Consciousness not only creates numerical data to depict patterns of preferences within this intrasocial group in the Dream Sociogram; it also elicits elaborations that prove very helpful to understand reality from the perspective of the group as a whole.

Designation of internal ambivalence

A final type of marking, mentioned above as a scoring of mixed preferences toward an element, involves the designation of *internal ambivalence*. There are times in your life when you are genuinely undecided. You are on the fence and have strong feelings pulling you in opposite directions. This is an authentic condition, although rarely a pleasant one. Consequently, there will be times when an interviewed character will experience genuine ambivalence toward a dream element. For instance, you may find that while your dream dog bites you for taking its bone and says it dislikes your action a lot (/2), it still feels genuine remorse because it basically loves you (3). In such a case, both positive and negative preferences are noted in one grid square. This would produce two scores in one box, in this case 3/2, or love and strong dislike. The positive preference is always written first. Other examples of double markings are: 1/1, 3/1, 2/3, 3/3, and 1/3.

Filling out the Dream Sociomatrix

In the example given above, *Ken Wilber Dies*, if this were your dream, you would begin by imagining that you are yourself back in it. Ask yourself, "How do I feel about myself in this dream? Do I like myself, like myself a lot, love myself, dislike myself, dislike myself a lot, or hate myself? Do I not feel one way or another? Do I feel a compassion toward myself that transcends all preferences? Do I feel some combination of feelings, such as strong like, yet dislike, or like, yet hatred?" Write the appropriate numerical designation, using the above numerical values, in the box where choosing Dream Self on the left column intersects chosen Dream Self on the top row. In the above example, Dream Self likes himself a lot in the dream, so a "2" is placed in the top-left box. This process is called *eliciting preferences*.

Any thoughts Dream Self has that explain his preferences are called *elaborations*. They are written in the Dream Sociomatrix Commentary. Next you ask yourself, as Dream Self, how you feel about the second chosen dream element, which in this case is "Ken Wilber." The preference "love," value (3), is numerically noted in the intersecting square and any elicited elaborations are written in the Dream Sociomatrix Commentary. This procedure is continued until Dream Self has expressed all of its preferences numerically in the appropriate squares toward all chosen dream elements and any associated elaborations are written in the Dream Sociomatrix Commentary.

You now move to the second choosing interviewed character, listed below Dream Self in the left-hand column. In this example, that interviewed character is "Ken Wilber." The same procedure is followed, continuing until all listed choosers have been given the opportunity to express their preferences numerically and provide elaborations for them. In this way, all listed choosing, interviewed characters are given the opportunity to express their preferences toward all chosen dream elements (characters, actions, and feelings) that are listed across the top of the Dream Sociomatrix.

Purpose of tabulation of preferences

The tabulation of interviewed character preferences provides you with a way to numerically describe the relative degree of acceptance or rejection different investid perspectives have toward themselves and others regarding the elements expressed in the dream/life drama. The importance of self-acceptance to self-development cannot be overstated. Recognizing how much you accept or reject yourself as well as understanding why and how you do so is fundamental to development. Preference tabulation also allows you to identify those perspectives both in conflict and supportive regarding those life issues that gave rise to a particular intrasocial group and to then depict these internal relationships in a Dream Sociogram. In addition, you will identify perspectives that you have ignored or misunderstood as well as those perspectives that are particularly competent in handling specific life situations that you encounter.

Location of the scores

The cumulative scores, which are the sums of both positive and negative preferences, are tabulated both on the right and bottom edges of the Dream Sociometric grid. You can see these totals in the Dream Sociomatrix example given above. Numbers on the *right* side of the grid represent totals added across the rows. Numbers on the *bottom* row represent totals added down the columns.

Tabulation of the scores

These totals, whether to the right or bottom, are first written as a ratio of the plus scores to the minus scores, with the positive score written to the left of the minus score in each pair: 6/14, for example. This means that there six degrees of positive preference and 14 degrees of negative preference were expressed.

An example of adding across a row from a different dream is found below from the Dream Sociomatrix for *Rescuing a Fish Out of Water*. There are cumulatively 21 positive degrees of preference and three negative degrees of preference (21/3) expressed by Dream Self. He liked three elements, liked nine elements a lot, and disliked one element. Notice that he did not love or hate any dream elements. He expressed neutrality toward one element, "Chest." There were no examples of internal ambivalence. The final number at the right, 18, is the sum of the plus and minus markings, making 21/3 the raw score for the interviewed character. Because row scores tabulate the scores of the preferring interviewed characters, they are listed on the acceptance axis of the Dream Sociogram, as we shall see.

Table 11.2

Dream Sociomatrix

Dream Date: 6/1/83
Name: Rescuing a Fish Out of Water

Smx Date: 6/3/83
Author: Dillard

	A.	B.	C.	D.	E.	F.	G.	H.	I.	J.	K.	L.	M.	N.	O.	CharAct Axis Totals	CharAct Raw Scores
	Dream Self	Inland	Fish	Alive	Pick up	Carry	Water	Breathe	* Unusual	No gills	Chest	Wiggled free	Lay quietly	Put in water	Hoped OK		
A. Dream Self	1	2	/1	2	2	2	2	2	1	-	1	/2	2	2	2	18	21/3
B. Fish	2	2	1	2	1/2	1/2	3	3	3	1	2	1	1	2	2	23	27/4
C. Inland	1	1	/1	1	1	1	1					/1	1	1	1	7	9/2
G. Water	1	1	/1	2	1	1	2	2	1	1	2	/1	1	2	2	14	16/2
K. Chest	1	1	1	2				2			2			2	2	12	12/0
El. Raw Scores	6/0	7/0	2/3	9/0	5/2	5/2	8/0	7/0	5/0	2/0	5/0	1/4	5/0	9/0	9/0		
El. Axis Totals	6	7	/1	9	3	3	8	7	5	2	5	/3	5	9	9		
El. Category	C	C	C	A	A	A	C	A	F	A	C	A	A	A	F		
Letter Name	A	B	C	D	E	F	G	H	I	J	K	L	M	N	O		

We can use the above example to explain adding down a column. For the first chosen element, at the top of the grid, there are six plus markings and no minus markings. The dreamer liked four interviewed characters and liked one interviewed character a lot. The final number at the bottom of the column, 6, is the sum of the plus and minus markings (of which there are none in this example), making 6 the column score for the dreamer. Because column scores tabulate the scores of all *chosen* elements (emotions and actions as well as interviewed characters), they must be listed from the choosing characters in the Dream Sociogram. Therefore, emotional element scores, noted with an asterisk at the bottom of the Dream Sociomatrix, are transcribed onto the affect, or emotional element axis of the Dream Sociogram. The action elements, designated with a dash at the bottom of the Dream Sociomatrix, are transcribed onto the process or action element axis of the Dream Sociogram. The chosen character scores at the bottom of the Dream Sociomatrix are transcribed onto the form or "perspective" axis of the Dream Sociogram. Unlike *row* totals, found to the right of the Dream Sociomatrix, which indicate *how accepting or rejecting one choosing interviewed character is toward all its fellow interviewed characters*, *column* totals indicate how preferring or rejecting *all* choosing interviewed characters are toward only *one* dream element.

Summary

- The Dream Sociomatrix is a device for objectifying preferences that exert significant but often largely unrecognized influence over what you do and how you feel.
- The Dream Sociomatrix collects numerical data based on preferences and elicits character elaborations that explain preferences.
- The assigning of numerical values to your preferences not only forces you to consider your feelings; it also provides a way to measure the interactional patterns among various invested and relatively autonomous perspectives.

Chapter 12

Obtaining interviewed dream character preferences

Learning how your choices create your reality

Wilson van Dusen has noted that

> Even a relatively stupid feeling out of one's own images is better than reason or the guess
> of the best outside experts. Outsiders are inclined to project their own lives into one's
> own images. Occasionally I have seen very good friends make meaningful guesses about
> another's images. But you are the life that projects your images. Your most halting under-
> standing is closer to its own source.

You interact with your environment based on the preferences you have moment
to moment. According to Viktor Frankl, "Man ultimately decides for himself!
And in the end, education must be education toward the ability to decide." The
more clearly and constructively you express your preferences, the less likely you
are to be controlled by your environment, by others and by internal factors
normally out of your awareness, such as early childhood script injunctions. The
problem is that most of your choices are subtle preferences that occur completely out of your awareness.

One of the benefits of Dream Sociometry is that it brings into awareness
preferences normally unrecognized that are determining your happiness so that
you can change the ones that aren't working for you. You will probably find
many instances in your dreams in which you express choices that are counterproductive. Don't be too hard on yourself about this, because this is normal and
a reality you will never outgrow because this process is intrinsic to development. Sometimes you yourself make these poor choices in the dream, as Dream
Self. In a dream called *Irresponsible House Parent*, Dream Self forgets to lock a
door and blames himself for youths running away who are under his care. Fear
reactions to monsters in nightmares are generally revealed to be another common example of poor dream choices by the dreamer. Unrecognized perspectives, represented as other interviewed characters, can also make poor choices.
In another dream called *Death in Flying Cars*, a character called "Boy" recklessly
endangers others and himself. The dream and action commentaries indicate

that sexual self-indulgence is viewed by this intrasocial group as thoughtless thrill-seeking. Often but not always, other characters that make poor choices are found to be surrogates for Dream Self, as revealed by similar patterns of preferences expressed as choosers in the Dream Sociomatrix.

Definition of element identification

As we have seen, a Dream Sociometric preference is obtained when an interviewed character states an opinion toward some element in the dream or life drama. When you identify with, or take the role of, an interviewed character in a dream narrative, a particular form of role- playing occurs called "*element identification*." J. L. Moreno pioneered a version of this role-playing procedure, and, as we have seen, it is an outgrowth of his sociometric methodology. Interviewed character preferences are elicited in order to understand both important interactions among stated preferences and their implications for your waking behavior. These interactions indicate behavioral patterns as well as attitudinal dynamics often out of your awareness. Preference patterns may also express the transpersonal perspectives that indicate how you can best align your life with the priorities of both your life compass and life itself.

How is it possible to "become" an interviewed character?

> *We are ensnared by the wisdom of the serpent; you are set free by the foolishness of God.*
> St. Augustine

Unlike St. Augustine, IDL sets aside prejudices against serpents and preferences for God. This is because we do not know, until they are interviewed, whether God and serpents are supportive or not. We may discover, for example, that God couldn't care less while the serpent is eager to help. This reasoning would itself be viewed as foolishness by St. Augustine because it questions the wisdom of a psychologically geocentrically determined reality. Instead, IDL says, "Why not create a collective reality, one that has the benefit not only of the preferences of waking identity, but of God, Serpents and whomever else happens along? If we are going to be divinely foolish, why not invite everyone and everything to the party?"

Some people wonder if an altered state is required in order to access the divine or transpersonal. The same question might be asked, "Is an altered state of consciousness required in order to quit watching TV and get up and take out the garbage?" Of course not! Then why do we need to access an altered state of consciousness to access the transpersonal? Both accomplishing the most mundane of activities and accessing the transpersonal involve shifts in role. You change roles constantly and spontaneously throughout the day without giving it a thought, yet we have seen how these states of consciousness may at times be extremely different when compared to each other. At one time of the day you may take care of the needs of a customer, while at another time, you take care of the sexual needs of your partner. These are very different roles, as you discover as soon as you imagine reversing them! What seems strange to you about identifying with interviewed characters is the fact that they are not only so concrete and unusual – chairs, cars, plants – objects you normally do not consider yourself to be, but so *mundane!* What's transpersonal about a chair? IDL and Dream Sociometry both demonstrate quite conclusively that this distinction is almost completely a delusion of our waking sense of self, one that is not shared by a majority of perspectives that you will interview.

To easily get into role, just consider God, serpents, and chairs as personifications of your waking roles, perspectives and feelings expressing themselves metaphorically as objects and as emerging potentials that are incarnating in drag, clown, and monster cartoons in order to wake you up so that you will listen to them![1]

You seamlessly shift state as you move from role to role throughout your day and even throughout your 24-hour waking-sleeping-dreaming cycle. Once you have experienced being a particular role, say a tree or a piece of plywood, you can identify with it whenever you want as easily as you might shift into the role of, say, consumer in a shopping mall. You can immediately get back into the unique perspective of this or that interviewed character whenever you want and just as easily flip back into your waking identity. There is no more of a sense of "possession" or "fragmentation" than you experience in the shift from traveler to reader.

Your awareness is dependent on the state you are in. Are you sleepy or alert? Are you numbed out or distracted by some addiction or clear and focused? Are you awake or asleep and dreaming? We generally assume that the state that we are in is the only one that is not "altered." It does not take the creation of too many Dream Sociograms to convince most people that from the collective perspective of interviewed intrasocial groups, *you* are the one with an altered consciousness! *They*, comprising not only the majority, but a collective *status quo*, is the new "normal" toward which you are headed. "Adjustment," then, is not successful adaptation to the expectations of family, school, peers, partners, work, and society, but to the shared cultural contexts generated by your intrasocial groups.

Identification with interviewed characters is not difficult, but it does require a certain amount of empathy. "Empathy" is an emotional identification with or vicarious experiencing of the feelings, thoughts, or perspectives of others. It basically requires a sense of self that is strong enough that it does not feel overwhelmed by experiencing the world from another perspective and a sense of self evolved enough to understand that it is in its own interest to do so.

Role playing or character identification is an entry level variety of empathy. Small children do it naturally. All that it requires is that you pretend that you are six again and imagine that you are a particular interviewed character, looking at the world through its eyes or from its perspective. The more you let yourself play at taking the roles of your interviewed characters the easier and more natural it will seem to become a dust pan, the opposite sex, God, or a squid. As you fill out the Dream Sociomatrix and express your preferences spontaneously, interviewed character identification soon becomes second nature.

While true empathy, the ability to see your world as others see it, does not generally arise until a child is at least seven or eight, the type of empathy that we are referring to here is almost innate. Almost every child can imagine that they are a mommy or daddy, a teacher, doctor, or soldier. Almost every child identifies with their dog or cat, even to the point of trying their food! Consequently, most people, excepting the most concretely character disordered or actively schizophrenic, can learn IDL. However, as is discussed in *Integral Deep Listening and Healing*, the inability to take the perspective of a dream character or the personification of a life issue is diagnostic. It may indicate not simply a reluctance or inexperience, but an actual inability to be empathetic, a disability that is associated with borderline, narcissistic and other personality disorders. Concomitantly, practice in imagining that you are this or that interviewed character cultivates the ability to empathize and is therefore not only inherently therapeutic but supports transpersonal development by defusing psychological geocentrism through the cultivation of multi-perspectivalism. As such, IDL promotes an expansion of self-identity without undermining whatever degree of "ego strength" a person already has.

Definition of a sociometric preference

A sociometric preference, within the context of IDL, is a feeling, perspective, or a perspective manifesting as a choice made by some interviewed character regarding a specific situation, individual, or concern. For example, if I say, "I like you," I am not simply stating a feeling. I am also expressing a perspective of receptivity and openness to someone I have yet to meet. I am also expressing a perspective that says, "Because we share an interest in Dream Sociometry we will probably enjoy each other's company." We can conclude that preferences are more than feelings, and choices are more than simple acts of will.

A preference is elicited from an interviewed character by taking on the identity of that interviewed character and asking yourself the sociometric question, "As interviewed character _____, how do I feel about (this element)?" For example, "As this cobra, how do I feel about this snake charmer? Do I like, greatly like, or love him? Do I dislike, greatly dislike, or hate him? Do I have no feeling about him one way or another?" Obviously, your unique response will be determined by many different factors: how thoroughly you take on the perspective of the cobra, your mindset at the particular time that you ask the question, the amount of time since you remembered the dream, and other factors.

Generally speaking, you will discover that you have both definite and even emphatic preferences as the cobra and that these preferences sometimes radically diverge from your own waking values and preferences. For instance, you might find this cobra saying, "I like this flute playing. It hypnotizes me. It takes my mind off of being stuck in that box all day." From this statement, the dreamer might conclude that *she* is feeling stuck in the box of her work all day and that she uses the hypnotic draw of sex to get release. By merely expressing such preferences, you will learn a great deal about yourself.

There are no "best" or "right" preferences

Different dreamers subjectively experience the worth and meaning of interviewed characters in different ways. Consequently, Dream Sociomatrix preferences are unique to each individual, reflecting personal criteria for evaluating each element. Does this mean that it is impossible to understand another person's intrasocial culture? On the contrary, sharing of sociomatrices, commentaries, and sociograms with partners, children, parents, and co-workers has been shown to be a powerful way to generate deeper respect, understanding, and compassion that translates into more patience and less drama in relationships.

The percentage of strong to weak preferences ("liking" to "loving," "disliking" to "hating,") will differ among dreams and among dreamers. There is no right or wrong, good or bad pattern of preference. All of us have had strong attractions that were destructive for us: jealous love, smoking, impulsive anger, and chronic sadness. This is the stuff great tragedies are made of, from *Oedipus Rex* and *Othello*, as well as the melodramatic wreckage of the average life. Similarly, you have strong dislikes which are often healthy, for instance, walking nude in snow, eating cigarette butts, or jumping into fire. Strong dislike, emotional neutrality, or strong attraction can all be highly productive, or they may result in tragedy. The *context* in which these preferences manifest determines their usefulness, and these contexts will be made abundantly clear in the commentaries.

The "best" and "right" preferences are those of the perspective stating its preferences! Remember this principle, because you will find that dreamers and students of IDL have a tendency to superimpose their interpretations not only on intrasocial groups but on themselves and each other. It is all too easy to forget that you are projecting your biases onto the experience of the interviewed emerging potential as well as the dreamer. This is a form of persecution within the Drama Triangle disguised as good-intentioned rescuing. There is, of course, a time and place for the projection of bias after the interviewed characters have been heard from and their contributions digested. However, when you are dropping your pearls of wisdom upon the dreamer, do not fool yourself by believing you understand their dream or life drama. If you remain silent and simply listen to what the dreamer tells herself in the guise of this or that interviewed character, you will learn much more than you will if you impress yourself by sharing your wonderful revelations about her experience.

Besides, there is not only no way to tell an interviewed character what preferences he or she should express, nor is there any good reason to do so. Your interviewed character preferences are real. They exist for important purposes. They deserve your respect and your thoughtful consideration. Your personal identification with your own interviewed characters and the stating of your spontaneous, honest preferences from its perspective provides the data that Dream Sociometry uses to help you heal, balance, and transform your life.

A comparison to the single-character interviewing protocol

The detailed and thorough nature of character identification is the greatest distinction between Dream Sociometry and the single-character interviewing dream and life issue protocols. While anyone can develop a series of questions to ask dream characters, the single-character interviewing protocol grows out of a method, Dream Sociometry, that uses a very thorough elicitation of the preferences of emerging potentials. Also, most questioning processes, including the single character interviewing protocol, do not collect preferences, give them numerical designations, or note them systematically. All of this *forces* the dreamer to get into role and stay in role in the absence of a questioner. This has obvious benefit for learning role identification, but what advantage does it provide for someone who is already able to shift into role quite easily?

The amount of information provided by emerging potentials by Dream Sociometry is typically much greater than in the single-character interviewing protocol not only because of the specificity of preferences and the clarity of the elaborations that are thereby elicited, but also because of the sheer number of elements that are considered. Consequently, Dream Sociometry provides much more in-depth practice in deep listening. It is normal in the single-character interviewing protocol to either ignore huge swaths of the dream or to make assumptions about what this or that non-interviewed character might have to say about it. Dream Sociometry leaves much less to chance. Dream Sociometry provides a way to provide answers without resorting to the self-satisfaction that rendering interpretations typically provides. While the single-character interviewing protocol reduces such tendencies, it is not nearly as effective at neutralizing them as is Dream Sociometry. Consequently, one of the fundamental advantages and purposes of creating Dream Sociomatrices is to teach your mind humility and the ability to reserve judgment, that is, take a phenomenological perspective, until relevant internal voices are heard.

Summary

- One of the perpetually amazing aspects of IDL is discovering how autonomous our inner preferences are. Exposure to them not only keeps us humble; it breaks down barriers between ourselves and the "other." This never stops, no matter how enlightened you become.

• Rather than leading to fragmentation or decompensation, identification with interviewed characters creates a broader, yet more secure sense of who you are.

• Dream Sociometry provides a very thorough form of both identification and elaboration of preferences.

Note

1 Of course, they are more than *waking* roles. They may be fixations or transpersonal potentials.

Chapter 13

Agreement in the Dream Sociomatrix

Agreement among preferring characters

This is indicated by the raw scores of choosing, or interviewed characters, found at the right margin of the Dream Sociomatrix. There are several different possible forms of agreement. Because preferences can be positive, negative, or neutral, agreement among preferring characters does not have to be positive. All choosers are in agreement in one or another of the following ways:

   highly preferring (raw scores like 15);
   preferring, to a greater or lesser extent (raw scores like 12 or 2);
   in conflict, which is an agreement to be confused (raw scores like 3/3, 10/9, 6/8, 4/7);
   neutral, meaning that none express any preferences whatsoever;
   rejecting, to a greater or lesser extent (raw scores like /7 or /3);
   highly rejecting (raw scores like /12 or /15).

A highly preferring score is determined by the number of possible preferences. In a small group a lower number, like 5 or /5 carries the same weight as a higher number, like 27 or /27, in a large group.

   Clearly, there are major implications, microcosmic, intrasocial, and psychological, on the one hand and macrocosmic, social, and globally systemic, on the other. These will be discussed in chapters that deal with understanding Dream Sociograms, where these relationships are laid out visually.

Agreement in expressing no preferences

Between 20% and 40% of the preferences in most Dream Sociomatrices in this series are neutral. Factors that influence this percentage include the investment of the dreamer in identifying with each interviewed character, the number of interviewed characters, and the number of dream elements. Longer Dream Sociomatrices tend to have more neutral preferences because there is a greater likelihood that some of the interviewed characters will not be invested in other segments of the dream in which they are not involved. Also, some life issues carry a stronger emotional charge than others, implying the expression of stronger preferences.

There is, of course, a distinction between having a preference and expressing it. It is quite normal to have preferences and to not express them. There can be several reasons for not doing so. The chooser may be unaware of his preferences, the chooser may be aware of a preference but misperceive its nature, or the chooser may simply choose not to express his preferences. Any of these alternatives could produce a relatively flat, low- preference Dream Sociomatrix. It is also possible that a dreamer could be actively working to suppress or neutralize his preferences. Centuries-old yogic and Eastern traditions advocate the elimination of desire because it is based on attachment to illusion and misperception. This type of individual might produce Dream Sociomatrices with fewer preferences, but I doubt it. I think if they were to fill out the Dream Sociomatrix honestly they would find that many preferences still exist, although they might well be much subtler than those of the average person.

Everyone has at least some opinions, perspectives, and preferences. Those that are associated with your various waking roles are the values that personify themselves as personal or emerging potentials that are persona surrogates. There exist other opinions, perspectives, and preferences that you do not know that you have until you interview emerging potentials. There is not only nothing wrong with having preferences; it is unhealthy not to have any at all, either due to denial, suppression, or perpetual transcendence. Eliminate *all* preferences, even those of your life compass, and you may succeed in eliminating most or all of your dreams. It is *attachment* to our preferences that creates suffering, not the inevitability of preference itself.

Consequently, almost every self-aspect, even doorknobs and asphalt roads, will usually be found to have definite opinions about something or somebody in its intrasocial environment. There are, however, different degrees of personal investment among self- aspects and among various intrasocial groups. Lack of preference generally indicates a prepersonal lack of empathy or a passivity on the part of the dreamer rather than transpersonal non-attachment. Non-attachment is often associated with a profound state of acceptance, known as *karuna* or "compassion" in Buddhism. As we have seen, IDL takes such "higher" preferences into account, although they are rare and, to the untrained, easily confused with having no preferences. On occasion, an absence of preferences may indicate some difficulty for the dreamer in identifying with various aspects of herself, as occurs in various personality disorders. If there exists a consistently high percentage of neutral responses by emerging potentials, a deep internal schism between intellect and affect may be present. This may not only be indicative of psychopathology; it may be possible to discriminate the type of psychopathology by the patterns of ambivalence that are observed in the Dream Sociogram.

Noting neutrality

Empty squares, counted as zero and representing neutrality, non-preference, non-choice, or disinterest are not counted, although they certainly represent a degree of preference. There are multiple possible motives for neutrality, and all of them are important. These run from unawareness, ignorance, and stupidity to highly aware objectivity and witnessing. Highly aware neutrality can be differentiated from normal, disinterested neutrality with a dot or some mark of your choice. It is also debatable as to whether this second variety can accurately be called "neutrality," as it represents the inclusion and transcendence of all preferences, including neutrality. If it is to be considered neutrality, then it is certainly a higher order or higher octave of neutrality from indifference.

It is possible to note the amount and percentage of neutrality of a particular chooser in his expressed preferences as well as the amount and percentage of neutrality received by each chosen element. These totals could be included as a separate score if the dreamer were interested in knowing the total degree of preference expressed by all choosers toward an element or how neutral a particular interviewed character is. These chooser neutrality scores could themselves be totaled for a sum of chooser neutrality, as a percentage of stated preferences. Similarly, the totals for neutrality scores of all chosen elements can be added for a sum of chosen element neutrality.

For instance, in a dream in which there are five interviewed characters and ten elements in all, there will be five choosers and ten chosen. At least 50 preferences will be expressed, more if there are instances of internal ambivalence, and for each preference, there are potentially seven degrees of preference. If one of the choosers expresses no preferences, each decision not to state a preference remains as significant as preferences themselves, because non-choice or indifference is itself a choice and a preference. While this tends to be represented as a low total of preferences both in the acceptance axis totals and on the acceptance axis placements in the Dream Sociogram, the data and where they come from are not explicit if neutrality is not totaled. If choosing characters are largely indifferent to some chosen elements but are highly preferring or rejecting of others, this is generally represented by high and low total scores and by similar relative Dream Sociogram placements on the relevant element axes. However, once again, neutrality totals are not explicit. In the examples in this text, specificity regarding neutrality totals is not noted, but it can be.

What is the significance of those Dream Sociomatrix patterns of preference that express a high degree of indifference in relationship to those that do not? A choice may be neutral due to a number of factors:

• Due to a lack of motivation to choose and a general indifference, an interviewed character may express a neutral preference. This is the typical motivation for a neutral preference, but it is important that it is not always the case.

- An interviewed character may prefer to remain neutral although he actually experiences some degree of attraction or rejection toward some interviewed character. If this is the case, it will be revealed in the Dream Sociomatrix Commentary, not in the numerical data.
- An interviewed character may state a neutral choice due to a lack of sufficient time to reflect and investigate the range of choices or because of a lack of information. This is neutrality due to ignorance.
- Ambivalence may result in a neutral choice, indicating confusion or conflict interior to the chooser. This source of neutrality is more likely to be found in Moreno's sociometry than it is in Dream Sociometry, because the expression of ambivalence by characters is encouraged and a means of doing so is readily available.
- An interviewed character may choose not to choose. Every now and then, an interviewed character may choose to disattach itself from the group. This is not indifference, ignorance, stupidity, or indifference, but neither does it imply idealism. Instead, it is most likely to be a rational calculation to avoid drama.
- The chooser may lack the ability to discriminate between a transcendent preference and a neutral one. For example, a chooser may base its neutral preference on high-level objectivity, witnessing, and empathy but not be able to differentiate that from indifference. This is much less likely than the opposite: assuming that indifference is transpersonal detachment, objectivity, empathy, and witnessing and thereby committing elevationism.
- A chooser may think that not choosing is a more powerful, less vulnerable position. This is a perspective commonly taken by a victim in the Drama Triangle.

Noting transpersonal neutrality

Complete acceptance is an extraordinary type of neutral "preference" that may from time to time be indicated by some of your interviewed characters. It is both rare and difficult to explain. It is indicated by grid squares that are marked with a dot, indicating the chooser's complete acceptance of both all preferences and no preferences regarding the particular chosen element. This experience transcends the six levels of preference, including that of love. Consequently, it can be perceived as compassionate, wise, or completely accepting. It is associated with witnessing, objectivity and a type of clear awareness that transcends dualities. It is transpersonal in that it is a relatively selfless choice. However, transpersonal neutrality is not noted in the Dream Sociogram. This is because it is not a numerical value, nor is it, strictly speaking, indicative of a degree of preference. While this type of acceptance in Dream Sociometry cannot be given a number and compared to degrees of preference, it can be counted, and those totals compared to preferences. That is, you can note a total sum of dots and compare who gives how many to whom and what elements receive so many dots.

While it may be argued that transpersonal acceptance is indeed a preference, it is most certainly not a preference in the same sense or order as the six preferences to which numerical values can be assigned. If the Dream Sociogram is a two-dimensional depiction of preferences, the seven values, including normal neutrality, can be placed in those two dimensions. Transpersonal neutrality or complete acceptance is in a third dimension. While its relationship to the other degrees of preference can be noted quantitatively, it is not strictly in the same plane of existence as the others.

An analogy can be made to the director of a play. Unlike the actors during performance and the audience, he does not view a murder with dislike or a romance with pleasure. He views both dispassionately, as artifices that are required in order to communicate the plot of the drama. This perspective is most likely to be observed in preferences expressed by Dream Consciousness, although it will generally express preferences. In fact, it was only with the inclusion of Dream Consciousness as a chooser that the category of transpersonal neutrality was discovered. Identification with such perspectives, when they do appear, cultivates detachment from the dramas of life and the unconscious. However, be aware that you may have a tendency to want to make your neutral scores or very strong positive ones into transpersonal neutrality, either due to an inability to discriminate among them due to the relative scarcity of experience with them, or because you want or hope to feel that way. Beware of a desire to be what you are not; this is a form of projecting your interpretations onto the perspective of this or that character, which means you are out of role.

Complete acceptance scores can be added not only as dots but as elaborations in the Dream Sociomatrix Commentary. For example, one could say, "Dream Consciousness expresses seven instances of transpersonal neutrality, Sky expresses four and broom expresses one." In this way, you could keep an account of those perspectives that express transpersonal neutrality under what circumstances and at what frequency.

Summary

- Dream groups that strongly prefer one another are generally highly positive, but there are notable exceptions, noted below.
- While intrasocial groups in which members strongly reject one another are conflictual, IDL generally experiences such conflict as highly positive.[1]
- Interviewed characters who express no preferences may be indifferent to the issue at hand, they may simply be emotionally dead, or they may be expressing a high order of witnessing and empathy. You can always ask them why they don't have many preferences.

- Dream Consciousness and some interviewed characters may on occasion report no preferences, yet clearly care a great deal. Such perspectives are both transcendent and transformative.

Note

1 There are various reasons for this, some of which are discussed in *Understanding the sociogram*. Antithesis is a natural and necessary stage of the developmental dialectic. Eliminate conflict, and you eliminate growth.

Bibliography

Dillard, J. (2018). *Understanding the sociogram.* New York: Routledge.

Chapter 14

Ambivalence in the Dream Sociomatrix

Ambivalence is conflict, cognitive dissonance, or indecisiveness expressed as a clash of preferences. It can be expressed toward one, many, or all dream elements. Ambivalence occurs in Dream Sociometry on the Dream Sociomatrix when two scores share one grid square in the Dream Sociomatrix. It is represented by a positive and a negative preference separated by a slash. Ambivalent raw scores can be seen at the right and bottom margins of the Dream Sociomatrix. While the distinction between neutrality and either positive or negative preferences can be considered a clash of preferences, the more common and stronger variety of ambivalence is between positive and negative preferences. There are four types of ambivalence and four degrees of ambivalence observed in the Dream Sociomatrix.

Four types of ambivalence

The four types of ambivalence found in the Dream Sociomatrix are Internal Ambivalence, Individual Ambivalence, Individual Internal Ambivalence, and Group Ambivalence.

Internal ambivalence

Occasionally, an interviewed character is so conflicted regarding his preferences toward a particular element that he cannot settle on only one degree of preference. Consequently, he feels both acceptance and rejection toward the same dream element. "Our greatest battles are those in our own minds," says Jameson Frank. Conjoining devas and asuras,[1] we project onto ourselves both attractive and repulsive characteristics. This is called *internal ambivalence* and is the first type of ambivalence found in the Dream Sociomatrix. It occurs when some choosing interviewed character both prefers and rejects some character, action or feeling. The score is written as some combination of positive and negative preferences in one grid square. Examples of such scores include 3/3, 3/2, 2/2, 2/3, 1/3, and 3/1.

Imagine that in a dream, you get angry at your pet dragon for torching your Christmas tree. Part of you likes a lot that you got angry because you feel justified. Besides, this is the third Christmas in a row that this has happened. Enough is enough. On the other hand, you know you reacted and lost control when you yelled at your dragon and you don't like that you yelled. After all, it was only doing what dragons do. Consequently, your score for the element anger would be 2/1. In another example, from the dream *Returning Golden Jewelry*, the interviewed character *Night* both likes and dislikes feeling *conspicuous* (1/1). *Night* is internally ambivalent regarding this particular emotion.

Internal ambivalence indicates that one particular aspect of a choosing perspective is in internal conflict regarding one particular aspect of the life issue that precipitated your dream or life drama. Notice that this is not the same as saying that this is a conflict within *yourself* or between two points of view within one of *your* roles. This is because, with the exception of Dream Self, who most definitely expresses conflicts within itself, *other characters* may be 1) parts of yourself, 2) not parts of yourself, 3) some combination of the two, or 4) neither. Do not make assumptions. When in doubt, ask them! Look for clarity in the commentaries! Generally speaking, unappreciated conflict constipates the ability to choose. It blocks the growth of your identity by creating preference barriers that not only separate you from yourself but internally divide emerging potentials, with the result that their presence, intention, and effect are less clear.

Summary of internal ambivalence

- Observed in the Dream Sociomatrix in individual scorings in grid boxes as chooser preferences.
- Involves the preferences of one choosing interviewed character.
- is indicated by both positive and negative preferences toward one element, whether character, action, or feeling.
- Indicates that an individual choosing interviewed character is conflicted in its preferences toward one chosen element.
- Technically, it can also involve conflict between neutrality and either preference or rejection.

Individual ambivalence

Individual ambivalence defined

Individual ambivalence occurs when a choosing character expresses positive preferences toward some chosen characters, actions or feelings and negative preferences toward others. Bertrand Russell has noted that "God and Satan alike are essentially human figures, the one a projection of ourselves, the other of our enemies." These aren't indicated in individual grid box preferences, but in raw totals at the right margin of the Dream Sociomatrix. When there is a mixed Character Raw Score total, mixed feelings exist within a *choosing* interviewed character toward the group of chosen elements. Individual ambivalence indicates that this or that chooser is experiencing internal conflict toward the intrasocial group *as a whole*. Consequently, that particular interviewed perspective is in conflict regarding how to address the issues concerning the group. It prefers some perspectives, actions, and feelings and rejects others. This results in some (+/−) combination in the character raw score totals at the right margin of the Dream Sociomatrix. These raw scores represent the sum total of individual ambivalence, or lack thereof, felt by that particular interviewed perspective toward *all* dream elements. Or, you could state only negative preferences toward all elements, which again would yield a non-conflictual raw score. Again, you could conclude that your critical and rejecting position was correct. Or, you could state only neutral preferences toward all elements, indicating that you have no preferences, don't care, or are indifferent, in most cases, or, extremely rarely, that you are transpersonally neutral.

Conversely, you may find a dream horrible and disgusting and hate every part of it, including yourself. Your character raw score is unambiguously negative. You cannot imagine that other parts of you could possibly disagree. However, when you interview other interviewed characters you find that some indeed *do* disagree, preferring what you hate. Just because you have no conflict in your preferences is hardly an indication that other perspectives will not have conflict either with you or within themselves. As you proceed to interview other perspectives, you will then be surprised to find that there are things about the situation that other characters do not like that you like and preferences that you make that other emerging potentials strenuously disagree with. Who is right? Who is wrong? Why don't they agree with *you?* Individual ambivalence records such internal conflicts and brings into stark clarity the assumptions behind your preferences. You come away from the experience with the conclusion that conflict and ambivalence are not bad things; on the contrary, they are wake-up calls.

A common waking analogy might be ambivalence about going for a walk. You may like the idea of getting exercise. At the same time, you may dislike the cold outside, creating some ambivalence toward sticking your nose out the door. You may prefer walking as an escape from a noisy house, yet at the same time, you may not like walking alone. As a result, you are internally conflicted about going for a walk. Now imagine that you were to ask your legs, your house, or your neighborhood how they felt about you going for a walk. Would they express the same pattern of ambivalence? Probably not! You can imagine that the more perspectives that have either internal or individual ambivalence, the more you are likely to be indecisive, confused, hesitant, and create barriers to your own growth. Your decision-making ability is going to suffer from such dissonance. This second type of Dream Sociomatrix ambivalence is called individual ambivalence because it emphasizes the conflict within this or that individual chooser toward the group as a whole.

While acceptance is on the whole associated with integration and congruence in Dream Sociometry, highly constructive intrasocial group elements are sometimes emphatically rejecting. For example, in the dream *The Hanging Corpse*, the *Old House* has a character raw score of 16/10, and the *Young Man* has a character raw score of 21/12. Both of these interviewed characters are highly accepting, as determined both by other preferences and by their elaborations and yet remain emphatically rejecting. Such rejection, when it is in the context of mixed raw scores, as these examples are, is always a statement of individual ambivalence.

Summary of individual ambivalence

- Observed in the Dream Sociomatrix and the Dream Sociogram
- Involves the preferences of one choosing character.
- Is indicated by character ratios at the right margin of the Dream Sociomatrix as raw scores.
- Indicates that a choosing character is conflicted in its preferences toward the group as a whole, preferring some and rejecting others.

Individual internal ambivalence

A special instance of this individual ambivalence occurs when the interviewed character is ambivalent toward *himself* in his preferences. Preferences of this sort, always expressed toward oneself, are mixed: 3/1, 3/3, 3/2, 2/1, 2/2, etc. Because self-criticism or lack of positive regard for oneself is inherently conflictual, any non-positive preference stated by a group member toward itself constitutes individual ambivalence. Any group whose members express a high degree of self-rejection and lack of self-acceptance is likely to be disturbing, if it is recalled or thought about at all. Such internal ambivalence is highly destructive and is probably the most important single aspect of the dynamics of the intrasocial group because it blocks the healing necessary for balance and transformation. Evaluation of the Dream Sociomatrix and Dream Sociogram needs to be directed toward answering such questions as: *why do these interviewed characters not like themselves? Why do I not like myself in this life situation? What can I do to like myself more in this life situation? If I cannot realistically like myself in this situation, how can I move toward a more neutral assessment of my role in this situation?*

Self-rejection by an interviewed character is always significant and indicates a denial of the worth of either some aspect of ourselves by ourselves or of some emerging potential. We are cutting ourselves off from a wake-up call, fire from heaven, or both. If you, as Dream Self, do not choose yourself, we know that the life issues reflected in the intrasocial group involve fundamental self-criticism and rejection by you of yourself. While it is not unusual to find ourselves disliking or hating various aspects of ourselves in our intrasocial universe, it is relatively rare in this sample to find these rejected aspects rejecting themselves as well. Usually, they will assert their self-worth and the importance of their cause. But when such emerging potentials condemn themselves there is a doubly damning process eating away at our psychic entrails, like hydrochloric acid creating ulcers. While such self-denial is not unusual among interviewed characters (each time a negative preference is stated this occurs, since all are in part projected aspects of self), *self*-rejection by an interviewed character is a particularly abominable form of self-condemnation.

Summary of individual internal ambivalence

- Occurs within interviewed characters as *choosers*
- Is observed only in the Dream Sociomatrix
- Involves individual preferences only
- Indicated by two numbers in the square indicating chooser self-preference.
- Indicates that the interviewed character is conflicted in its preferences toward itself
- Creates positive-negative acceptance ratios in raw scores at the right margin of the Dream Sociomatrix.

Group ambivalence

If there is no struggle there is no progress.

Frederick Douglass

Group ambivalence defined

Most growth happens out of awareness, without any experience of struggle. In addition, much stress is productive, or eustress, leaving only a relatively small residue for most of us, most of the time, that is experienced as struggle. However, when struggle feels real to us, the best response is to face into it and work through it and this is what you are doing when you confront ambivalence in Dream Sociometry. The fourth type of ambivalence in the Dream Sociomatrix, *group ambivalence*, occurs when one chooser disagrees with another in his or her preferences toward the same chosen character, action, or feeling. Group ambivalence is expressed as the ratio of positive to negative preference scores at the *bottom* margin of the Dream Sociomatrix. This indicates that the characters that you are interviewing in this particular dream or life drama do not agree with each other about how they feel toward some perspective, action, or feeling that you hold. This type of conflict is relatively broad-based, in that it concerns all choosers, but is yet specifically focused, in that the group is in conflict regarding one specific character, action, or feeling. Of course, the more elements that are the objects of group ambivalence, the more pervasive is the internal conflict. This type of Dream Sociomatrix ambivalence is called *Group Ambivalence* because it emphasizes the conflict within the intrasocial group as a whole toward this or that dream element. In contrast, individual ambivalence is limited to this or that choosing aspect of yourself, yet expressed broadly toward the group as a whole.

Since group ambivalence exists within a group of interviewed characters when they are divided in their preferences toward one element, it is expressed as both like and dislike toward some dream element in the preference scores at the bottom of the Dream Sociomatrix. For instance, such raw scores as 7/3, 2/2, 2/9, 1/6, and 5/5 appearing at the bottom of the Dream Sociomatrix indicate group ambivalence. In such a case, mixed feelings toward the element exist among choosing interviewed characters. For example, in the dream, *Never Eat Possum*, five interviewed characters like that Possum is *no good to eat*, while three dislike it. The raw score of 9/6 given *no good to eat* indicates that the intrasocial group experiences moderate ambivalence toward this interviewed character.

Element ratios (the column scores found at the bottom margin of the Dream Sociomatrix) indicate the extent to which choosing interviewed characters are in agreement regarding how they feel toward a particular dream element. Strong agreement and a high raw preference ratio indicate strong internal congruence among interviewed characters toward a particular perspective. It also indicates low ambivalence. For instance, in the dream *Spider in the Car, Family, Car*, and *Rear-View Mirror* all have element raw scores that indicate strong group member agreement and a high raw preference ratio. Low agreement and a high raw preference ratio indicate strong group ambivalence among interviewed characters toward this particular aspect of self. For example, in *Spider in the Car, Back Seat* has an element raw score of 7/8, indicating low agreement among interviewed characters and a high raw preference ratio.

Ambivalence may also be observed in some interviewed character elaborations in the Dream Sociomatrix Commentary.

Summary of group ambivalence

- Observed in the Dream Sociomatrix and the Dream Sociogram
- Involves positive and negative preferences in the collective preferences of *choosing* interviewed characters.
- Is indicated by element ratios at the *bottom* of the Dream Sociomatrix
- Indicates that the group of choosing interviewed characters is divided in their preferences toward a chosen element.

Degrees of ambivalence

It is well to remember that while the elimination of internal conflict is generally advocated by interviewed characters, growth does not occur without it. Generally speaking, the more ambivalence that is experienced in life, whether within a intrasocial group or within waking experience, the more opportunities for growth exist. As Irma Bombeck has said, "The grass is always greenest over the septic tank." For example, the antithesis stage of every developmental process presupposes conflict; the transformation exemplified by synthesis presupposes the healthy navigation of a previous antithetical stage. Consequently, it is wise to focus on managing and maximizing the positive aspects of conflict rather than attempting to eliminate it. However, too many strong conflicts at the same time can be overwhelming. Dream Sociometry makes such an onslaught less likely by bringing conflicts to the surface before they reach alarming proportions on multiple fronts. The four degrees of ambivalence observed in the Dream Sociogram are low, moderate, high, and direct. Less ambivalence means less internal conflict. More ambivalence means more internal conflict.

Ambivalence can express conflict between yourself and other roles you consciously take, as occurs in smokers between smoking and not smoking. It can express conflict between yourself and roles you possess but don't consciously take, as between a self-image that says you are kind and thoughtful and your uncontrolled temper. Ambivalence can also express conflict between yourself and unrecognized, unborn emerging potentials. These are perspectives that are not yet part of your self definition but are trying to be. Look to the elaborations in the various commentaries to determine which of these possibilities you are dealing with.

In the case of individual ambivalence, while the choosing interviewed character is unlikely to see itself as being abusive in its preferences, *rejected* interviewed characters may have a different opinion, as may other interviewed characters toward whom no preference is expressed. In the case of group ambivalence, while there are notable exceptions, it is not unusual for interviewed characters to state that they do not like being the subject of such group conflict.

Low ambivalence

Low ambivalence exists in the Dream Sociomatrix when any acceptance or element raw score ratio is less than 40% but above 0%, in which case, ambivalence would not exist at all. To arrive at this ratio, the lower number is divided into the higher. Here are some examples of low raw score ratios: 5/2, 2/8, and 3/11.

Such scores indicate relatively low levels of conflict within the individual choosing interviewed character (acceptance raw scores) or within the intrasocial group as a whole (element raw scores). Of course, other interviewed characters can at the same time express high degrees of ambivalence toward some other dream elements. Because there is general interviewed character concurrence in how the element is viewed, these elements receiving low ambivalence scores tend to support the group *status quo*. If the group homeostasis is healthy, such support can be helpful. But the group stasis may be destructive, severely retarded, or rigid, making the benefit of such support highly questionable. For instance, most element raw scores in the dream *Death in Flying Cars* exhibit little or no ambivalence. This indicates a surprising degree of passive acceptance of destructive internal dynamics by this congregation of invested perspectives.

Low ambivalence for totals in which few preferences are expressed, such as 3/1 and 4/1, are often not noted in this sample because there is not enough conflict indicated to be particularly significant.

Moderate ambivalence

Moderate ambivalence exists in the Dream Sociomatrix when any acceptance or element raw score ratio is 40% or more and less than 70%. Examples are 3/2, 2/1, 9/6, 4/2, and 15/21.

Such scores indicate moderate levels of conflict by a choosing interviewed character (acceptance raw score) or within the group as a whole regarding preferences toward some dream element (element raw score). Such an element is perceived as a significant obstacle or irritation to one or more interviewed characters. We cannot conclude from this that the element is inherently obstructionist; some portion of another intrasocial group might not perceive it so much as an obstacle but rather as simply distasteful, scoring low ambivalence, or it might even be highly preferred. In a nightmare antithetical pattern, an element may be preferred that would be rejected by other intrasocial groups (say a bloody knife or an ax murderer). Sometimes, elements are rejected because subgroups feel threatened by them.

In any case, it is well to remember that rejected interviewed characters are aspects of self or potential aspects of self that are being disowned. While such a choice is sometimes appropriate, rejection usually occurs in a knee-jerk, reactive fashion without sufficient consideration. While it is theoretically possible (I am reminded of Krishna advising Arjuna to slay his relatives in the *Bhagavad Gita)*, rarely is it undertaken from a truly transpersonal perspective. The significance of moderate ambivalence can easily be overshadowed and overlooked in favor of the more intense conflicts reflected by higher ambivalence scores. But a series of moderate ambivalence scores may carry the combined potency of one or two very high scores. In addition, a score of 7/15 may indicate a more significant conflict than a score indicating low-level direct ambivalence, such as 2/2, simply because more aspects of self are divided against one another (in the case of element axis ambivalence). More intention is invested in the conflict. It is also important to remember that in some dreams there is very little ambivalence. That may indicate that low or moderate ambivalence scores carry the same significance for that particular group that high ambivalence carries for more conflicted groups.

High ambivalence

High ambivalence exists in the Dream Sociomatrix when any acceptance or interviewed character raw score ratio is 70% or more and less than 100%. Examples: 4/3, 11/9, 8/7, 22/26. Note that it is not possible to have high ambivalence for those elements that receive very few preferences since a score like 2/3 indicates moderate ambivalence and 3/3 indicates direct ambivalence.

High ambivalence scores indicate either significant levels of conflict within one interviewed character toward the group as a whole (individual ambivalence) or within the group as a whole regarding its preferences toward one element (group ambivalence). In the former case, the energies of one specific interviewed character are being drained away from the group by its fixation on perceived conflict. In the latter case, such an element becomes a focal point of the group's attention, drawing its energies to it like some microcosmic black hole. Consequently, these elements receive attention that provides them with inflated importance in relation to other elements. It is doubtful that they are actually any more important than any other element, but because the group members *perceive* them as particularly important, other business must be laid aside while the issues pertinent to that element and its relationship to the group are first addressed.

We have seen how it is impossible to construct a dreamage when no conflict resolution regarding one or more of such elements is possible. This underscores the significant potency of those elements receiving highly ambivalent preferences. They can stop growth dead in its tracks. Clearly, it is important that the role of such an element in the intrasocial dynamics of the group be understood if its disruptive influence in waking and dream awareness is to be redirected. Pay particular attention to the Action Commentary suggestions made by these elements.

Direct ambivalence

Direct ambivalence exists in the Dream Sociomatrix when any raw score ratio displays the same number of positive and negative preferences. Examples: 3/3, 11/11, 8/8, 22/22. Obviously, low scores are not only more common than high ones, but can signify a smaller amount of life force tied up in conflict, making a score of 9/9 much more significant than say, 2/2. Of course, the size of the group matters. If you have three choosers and seven elements, it is impossible to highly score any type of ambivalence at all. Therefore, a score of 2/2 in a small group could represent as much intrasocial conflict as a score of 20/20 in a large one.

To the extent that character and group ambivalence imply self-abuse, direct ambivalence implies significant self-abuse. For example, Dream Self in the dream *Dad Dies*, a intrasocial group not included in this series, experiences a very high degree of direct ambivalence: 23/23. In the same intrasocial group, *Father* experiences 17/17. The nature of this conflict is amplified and clarified in their Dream Sociomatrix Commentary elaborations. *Family*, in the dream *Death in Flying Cars*, experiences a great deal of ambivalence (9/9). (Note that there is often little group conflict toward an interviewed character expressing high or direct ambivalence, such as this one. The interviewed character *Family* was not disliked by any interviewed characters.)

Remarks made regarding high ambivalence bear repeating here, but more emphatically: such scores indicate extreme levels of conflict within the group regarding its preferences toward some element. If ambivalence indicates self at war, then direct ambivalence is the internal equivalent of Picket's Ridge at Gettysburg, the Israeli- Palestinian war, or the implosion of Yugoslavia: there are no real winners, only losers. The element is a serious obstacle for many if not all members of the group, and it is essential that its place in the dynamics of the group be understood if its disruptive influence in waking and intrasocial awareness is to be reduced. Normally, these conflicts go unattended and in one way or another work themselves into the fabric of personality, either as overt behaviors, misperceptions and emotional upsets, or as covert wounds or fixations that sap energy, slow down physical healing by increasing the amount of resistance and interior stress and distract from efforts to balance and transform. We adapt and go on, but we are the walking wounded.

Is direct ambivalence really that much more significant than high ambivalence? An element or two can easily be left out of the Dream Sociomatrix when it was created, creating direct ambivalence, or the lack of it "by accident." If those elements had been included, direct ambivalence probably would no longer exist. Similarly, if the Dream Sociomatrix had been created at a different time, the pattern of preferences expressed would probably have been somewhat different. Direct ambivalence is rather arbitrary, in that the addition or subtraction of one element from the dream or life drama would probably change direct ambivalence to high ambivalence. Therefore, the important point is that it indicates a lot of intense, serious disagreement and therefore some type of constipation.

Nevertheless, preference tendencies are fairly stable over time, meaning that if an interviewed character hates some element today, it is unlikely to love it in five years. While it is appropriate not to indulge too heavily in the significance of a case of direct ambivalence, it should hardly be ignored, particularly when several cases manifest in one and the same Dream Sociomatrix. Direct ambivalence is simply an emphatic statement of the intensity of some unresolved inner issue. Centrifugal and centripetal intrasocial forces converge and counterbalance each other creating an "energy knot" which makes conflict resolution of related life issues that much more difficult. Treat cases of intense high ambivalence, such as 9/10, 19/18, in a similar way.

Summary

Internal Ambivalence:

> One chooser both prefers and rejects one character, action or feeling. Found in individual scoring boxes. Indicates that one chooser is experiencing internal conflict toward some feeling, action, or perspective.

Individual Ambivalence:

> One chooser both prefers and rejects different chosen dream elements. Found in character raw scores at the right margin of the Dream Sociomatrix. Indicates that this self aspect is experiencing internal conflict toward the intrasocial group as a whole.

Internal Individual Ambivalence:

> One chooser both prefers and rejects *himself.* Found in the intersecting grid square of same choosing and chosen intrasocial group member. Indicates strong internal conflict within a specific interviewed character.

Group Ambivalence:

> All choosers both prefer and reject one dream element. Found in element raw scores at the bottom margin of the Dream Sociomatrix. Indicates that interviewed emerging potentials are in conflict toward some feeling, action, or perspective.
> • While the intensity of ambivalence generally indicates greater internal conflict, such conflict is not necessarily harmful or to be eliminated. This is determined by the context in which the conflict is occurring. Examination of both the Dream Sociogram as a whole and the pattern in the context of other Dream Sociograms will help you to arrive at a healthy assessment.

Note

1 Gods and demons of Hinduism.

Chapter 15

Interviewed character categories and attributes

> *To get to the core of God at his greatest one must first get into the core of himself at his least, for no one can know God who has not first known himself.*
>
> Meister Eckhard

Characteristics of elements

> *The world . . . is only beginning to see that the wealth of a nation consists more than in anything else in the number of superior men that it harbors.*
>
> William James

Our worth consists in good measure of the number of wise and nurturing perspectives that we access, without and within. There exist four basic preference extremes expressed by interviewed characters, most accepting, most rejecting, most preferred, and most rejected. They are called extremes because they are not average preferences. Choosing interviewed characters lie somewhere on a continuum from most accepting to most rejecting. Their placement is determined by their preferences. Chosen dream elements lie somewhere on a continuum from most preferred to most rejected. These categories identify the elements, whether choosing characters or chosen characters, actions, and feelings, that are at the ends of these continua. In addition, non-invested choosers express no preferences. Chosen elements may be isolates, with few, if any, preferences expressed toward them.

Most accepting

Surprisingly, natural and inanimate elements that rarely have a central role in a dream are often the most accepting of their fellows. Perhaps their relative noninvolvement allows them to observe issues with detachment and objectivity without reacting to the situation. Non-human interviewed characters are typically more accepting than the average human interviewed character. This most likely is due to our relative identification with humans, which results in heightened projection of feelings and motivations. Vehicles, houses, and buildings are often more accepting than their human occupants. In fact, the more "different" an interviewed character is from waking awareness, the more accepting it seems to be. Again, this seems to relate to our waking identifications and how they tend to exclude and discount perspectives that are unlike our own.

Accepting characters express more positive preferences than negative ones. They love, like a lot, or like more elements than they dislike, dislike a lot, hate, or feel neutral about. However, a character can be critical and negative, expressing few positive preferences and still qualify as the most accepting member of a highly rejecting group. In addition, the most accepting character may be the most destructive or abusive. Imagine a group of thugs. Those who are the most violent and abusive get the most praise and respect from their peers.

Most rejecting

In many instances, Dream Self or some Dream Self surrogate is the most rejecting character in a dream. A Dream Self surrogate is a character whose preferences are similar to those of Dream Self. This explains some nightmare patterns, when we are shocked to find that the intrasocial group as a whole sees us essentially the same as the enemy we fear. I am reminded of the terrible old pun, "When two egotists meet, it's an I for an I."

In IDL, waking identity usually ends up being the aspect of awareness that needs to take remedial classes in acceptance and nurturance. It can be humiliating to discover that a brick wall or some nasty goblin is more accepting than you are. Dream Self and its surrogates are often discovered to be the most closed and the most defensive members of the group, not the monster, spider, killer, or other perceived antagonists. If you find this to be the case for your intrasocial groups, what does this say about your ability to make healthy decisions about yourself and others in your waking life? A useful conclusion is, "I will probably make better decisions if I consult intrasocial perspectives that take broader perspectives and are healthier than I am." Character identification tends to instill a great deal more humility and caution in making habitual waking decisions.

Remember that normally nurturing perspectives can and will express the most negative preferences if bad things are happening and they don't like them. This is what happens in nightmare antithesis patterns.[1] Just as the most accepting interviewed characters are not necessarily those that express the most positive preferences, so the most rejecting perspectives are not necessarily those that express the most negative preferences. Context creates meaning. Change the context, change reality.

Most preferred

Those elements that are most preferred are known as "stars," following Moreno's usage. Every group has a most preferred character, action and feeling. Even if a group were to contain only rejected elements, those that were least rejected would be most preferred by the group. In addition, a character's feelings may be rejected by a group, while his actions and identity are accepted. His actions may be rejected, while his feelings and identity are accepted.

A character is not necessarily wise or nurturing just because he is most preferred by the intrasocial group, since the group itself may be dominated by abusive perspectives. Generally, however, those characters that are most preferred by the group are the sociometric stars because they are most preferring. If you respect their needs, you gain the respect of the group. If you ignore their needs, you will probably isolate the entire group. In those groups in which Dream Self is the most preferred character, in effect *you* are the sociometric star. This means that your perspectives, actions, or feelings are most preferred by that particular group, for better or for worse. This can come as a shock. You may be surprised to see yourself preferred by self-destructive perspectives. You may find yourself in the awkward position of being placed in a position of responsibility in relationship to other perspectives, a position you didn't seek and don't feel comfortable with. If you persevere with IDL, you will find this sort of relationship with your characters showing up more and more frequently. How will you respond when you discover that you are looked up to by perspectives and seen as their savior?

Most rejected

Highly rejected elements are perspectives that indicate where you are stuck. They are in pain and need to be listened to particularly closely. Sociometrically, those elements which are most rejected by the choosers are known as "rejects." While highly rejected elements are generally dysfunctional, they are always an important part of your life that has in some way come into conflict with other parts. Healthy perspectives can and do get rejected. When you practice deep listening to highly rejected perspectives, you incorporate into your identity those components of your *élan vital* that have previously existed out of your awareness or in your awareness but misperceived.

Dream Self and its surrogates are often accepted while their feelings and actions may not be. Interviewed characters make a distinction that we often forget in our waking lives: to hate the evil deed but to love the person; to differentiate between feelings and actions on the one hand and beingness on the other. If you learn this one bit of wisdom from your encounter with your intrasocial universe, you have learned a great deal.

Non-invested interviewed characters

Non-invested interviewed characters express few preferences. The few that are stated are minimal, an occasional like or dislike, no more. This non-investment may be a statement of indifference or it may be an expression of non-attached transpersonal neutrality. You can determine which by the character's elaborations in the Dream Sociomatrix Commentary. If the non-investment of a character is due to indifference, their comments will reflect both a lack of energy and relationship. Do not, however, assume that they are irrelevant to the dynamics of the group. They may personify important perspectives that need to become invested in order for the group to attain balance. They may also be highly preferred by members of the group despite their own lack of investment. If this is so, other characters will prefer them, and you will probably find these preferences explained in the elaborations. If the non-investment of a character is due to non-attachment, their elaborations are likely to display one or more of the following: considerable energy, awareness, acceptance, wisdom, equanimity, confidence, and compassion. The character is simply not choosing to express these qualities through preferring. This is a relatively enlightened perspective. It is the reason the non-numeric preference "transcending all preferences" is included as an option in creating the Dream Sociomatrix.

Isolates

Isolates are elements that receive few, if any, preferences. Clearly, these elements are at a polar extreme from those elements that are both highly preferred and highly rejected *at the same time*. These may superficially look similar, in that they both have low axis totals and are placed at or very close to the center of the Dream Sociogram. There is a tremendous difference between them, however. While isolates are ignored, elements that are both highly preferred and highly rejected at the same time are obviously the objects of intense character feelings.

While isolates are largely ignored by their fellows, they themselves may express strong preferences which are both relevant and helpful. Like non-invested characters, isolates that express few preferences are either non-invested perspectives lacking life or direction or non-attached perspectives that exist above the fray.

In either case, isolates are perspectives that are essentially ignored by the group. Does this mean that they are unimportant? It may be that they are indeed unimportant to this group, yet the group has overlooked qualities or characteristics that are important, just as we sometimes do in our waking life. It is easy to get so focused in on an issue that we ignore important information or help that we need. Dream sociometric groups can also do this. To discover whether or not this is the case, consider the elaborations of the isolate. Are they disinterested, or are they indicative of perspectives and interests that are beneficial to the group?

Character attributes

Can you imagine driving along, looking in your rearview mirror and discovering, to your horror, that there is a gigantic black spider in the back seat? No wonder you repress your dreams! This is a situation where fear exists and hope does not – at least not in that first reaction! But, when the *Spider* is interviewed in the dream *Spider in the Car*, Dream Self starts to become aware of how he scares himself to add drama to his life. *Spider* says, "I like the car and family because they are potential victims." This is scary enough. But he goes on to say, "I put on a good show, keep things moving." It's hard to be too scared of someone whose main purpose in life is to relieve you of your boredom. When you acknowledge the existence and perspective of interviewed characters, particularly those that seem most vile to you, you come to understand yourself, even at your worst and, at the same time, discover there is no place where hope is not.

While some interviewed characters may exemplify egotism or prepersonal ethical development and others echo the perspectives, feelings, and behaviors of the dreamer, you will often encounter voices that express opinions and hold perspectives that are relatively objective, accepting, and non-reactive when compared to those held by you. This is determined not only by the different patterns of preferences in the Dream Sociomatrix, but by the reasons and motivations behind the statements made in the various commentaries. The fact that we can have easy and available access to emerging potentials is not merely important; it is a major source of support and direction for the evolution of human consciousness. If there exist perspectives readily available to you that express preferences that are relatively objective, mindful, accepting, and non-reactive when compared to those you hold, what implications might we draw? Here are several possibilities:

- Regardless of your level of development, you are likely to encounter a good number of interviewed perspectives who are more evolved than you are on one or more developmental line.
- Your identification with more evolved emerging potentials is likely to speed your development.
- Because these perspectives are not born, they cannot die. Therefore, they are not motivated by the same fears of death that you and I are.
- Because they are less invested in fear, particularly fear of death, they are likely to be less attached, more detached, and more objective than you are.
- Consequently, these relatively secure emerging potentials are more likely to handle the stress and suffering in your life better than you do.
- They are less likely to be afraid of others than you and I are because they cannot be killed. Having no possessions, they possess nothing to steal.
- They are more likely to manifest attributes of the transpersonal, particularly your life compass.

Here is a description of some of the more significant characteristics observed in a majority of those interviewed characters whose patterns of preferences are more accepting than those of Dream Self:

Relative autonomy

There is no guarantee that any particular interviewed character or intrasocial group will support your wishes and desires. In fact, you may be disgusted by what some interviewed characters have to say. In *Equine Cannibals*, *Three Horses* say that they have no ethics. They'll eat whatever they can get, including another horse. This kind of statement forces the dreamer to consider when and how he surrenders his ethical standards and, in the process, devours himself. In acknowledging the relative autonomy of his destructiveness, he begins to reclaim and reintegrate it into an expanded sense of self.

You will experience the relative autonomy of your interviewed characters for yourself when you interview them. The experience of this autonomy is basically a function of your willingness to let go of your waking sense of self and identify with different perspectives. The more successful you are at doing so, the more likely you are to experience an amazing degree of autonomy that will make you question the origin of these perspectives. To say that they are a part of you is to expand your identity to include not only things you disagree with but with potentials that you have not yet begun to recognize, that are only now being birthed within you.

You will find that interviewed perspectives may or may not agree with you and may or may not support your cherished opinions, beliefs, and preferences. The relative autonomy of your interviewed characters creates a surprising objectivity in a realm that many expect to provide the epitome of subjectivity. When we stop to think about this, it is reductionistic to claim that such objectivity and autonomy is a part of ourselves. It both makes us bigger than we are, in a statement of narcissistic grandiosity, while reducing emerging potentials to a mere facet of ourselves. The basic rationale for claiming ownership of interviewed perspectives is to teach responsibility and withdraw projections. It is to avoid committing the mistake of disownership intrinsic to shamanism, magic, spiritualism, and New Age channeling.

People conclude that they must do one or the other rather than practicing deep listening in an integral way to these perspectives themselves and sitting at the foot of their wisdom. When you do you may discover what others have, that they partially belong to you and are partially do not, partially subjective and objective and yet are neither. This is because they are living, vibrant expressions of what it means to be a holon, a part-whole that is both individual and collective, interior and exterior, self and other, irreducible to either.

Interviewing such perspectives is an experiential antidote to the prevailing tendency of science to discount inner consciousness as mere subjectivity, as psychology did when it steered away from Wunch and phenomenology in order to establish its credentials as an objective science. The objectivity that you will encounter in these perspectives is a consistently present and self-correcting tool for learning to watch yourself go by and for discovering your blind spots. In both of these ways, it proves itself to be a vital adjunct to guidance from peers, professionals and social norms.

While there is nothing inherently transpersonal about relative autonomy, there is a tendency for this autonomy to increase as you thin your sense of self. While the independence of adulthood is clearly more autonomous than the dependency of childhood, it is less obvious that the interdependence of maturity is more autonomous than independence. This is understood when we remember that autonomy grows based on our willingness to expand our identity, to incorporate into ourselves the interests and perspectives of others without fear of overwhelm or loss of self. Setting ourselves apart from others is not nearly as autonomous a position as setting ourselves within the context of others, yet remaining ourselves. In this regard, relative autonomy is a hallmark of both interdependent co-origination and a transpersonal approach to life.

Acceptance

The acceptance of others and self-acceptance are one in the same from the perspective of IDL. This is because the process of IDL interviewing is instruction in the experience that when you accept interviewed characters by becoming them and listen respectfully to what they say, you are accepting those perspectives, roles, and preferences within yourself that they personify; to reject interviewed characters is merely to reject yourself, which means to generate greater conflict within yourself. Is that wise? Who would want to do that? IDL provides experiences demonstrating that it is practical, logical, and beneficial to treat others as you wish to be treated. This is because, from the perspective of IDL there is no psychological difference between self-acceptance and acceptance of others, since others are phenomenologically aspects of ourselves. A little personal and direct experience of this fundamental truth is much more effective than years of moralistic education.

A consistent and fascinating characteristic of many interviewed characters is their willingness to unconditionally accept you at those times and in ways when you will not accept yourself. If you value the cultivation of self-acceptance, I know of no source that provides the experience of genuine and deep acceptance as consistently as does IDL.

What is it about acceptance that is so important to development into the transpersonal? Acceptance assumes both trust and respect. It is impossible to be truly accepting when fearful. While we may acquiesce or agree to reduce our fear, this hardly qualifies as acceptance. The absence of acceptance, whether of self or others, implies separation. Separation, if maintained, supports dualism rather than unity. It might fairly be said that meditation, widely viewed as the core transpersonal practice, is itself a practice of the cultivation of acceptance. In meditation, thoughts, sensations, and feelings are all observed with equanimity and acceptance.

You will find that many of your interviewed characters are more accepting than you are. Test this assumption by simply asking yourself how accepting you consider yourself to have been, on the average, during the past week, on a scale of zero to ten, with zero being very unaccepting and ten being extremely accepting of yourself and others. Next, ask a few of your previously interviewed characters how accepting *they* are. If you find that many of your interviewed characters are more accepting than you are, this implies that they deserve your respect.

Wisdom

Wisdom is the right application of knowledge. A person can be smart and not wise. Similarly, a person can be dumb, in that they lack intelligence, or ignorant, in that they lack knowledge, yet still be wise if they possess an innate wisdom that guides their actions. If a person does a good job of applying the knowledge that they do have, they can be wise even if they lack the knowledge that most people consider to be required for both wisdom and success. Forrest Gump, the lead character in the movie of the same name, is an excellent example of this attribute.

You will probably find that a majority of your interviewed characters are wiser than you are. Test this assumption by simply asking yourself how wise you have been, on the average, during the past week, on a scale of zero to ten, with zero being very unaccepting and ten extremely wise. Next, ask a few of your interviewed characters how wise they are. If you find that many of your interviewed characters are wiser than you are, doesn't this imply that they are worth listening to?

Empathy

While love is generally a strong and personal emotion, compassion is neither emotional nor personal, although it can most certainly be strong. Empathy is a selfless and relatively impersonal and altruistic respect which is not a feeling or motivated by feeling, as are compassion and sympathy. Interviewed characters are innately empathetic in that they know you at least as well as you know yourself, if not better.

As with wisdom, you will find that while few may state preferences that transcend love, many will prove themselves by their preferences to be more empathetic than you are. You can perform the same experiment with empathy that you did with wisdom to demonstrate this to your own satisfaction. If you desire to grow your love into empathy, you can do worse than to practice identifying with those perspectives that demonstrate more empathy than you do.

Equanimity

Equanimity is peace of mind. If you are rich but don't have peace of mind, you won't enjoy your wealth. If you are healthy but don't have peace of mind, you can't enjoy your health. If you are loved and adored by all but don't have peace of mind, the approval of the masses will mean little to you. Consequently, the attainment and maintenance of peace of mind is fundamental to happiness. It is indeed a priority of your life compass.

You can decide for yourself if equanimity is a priority of your life compass by asking your interviewed characters how much peace of mind they possess. You can also determine if the majority of your interviewed characters have more peace of mind than you do by conducting the above experiment with them. This implies that practicing deep listening to your interviewed characters is an effective path leading to the cultivation of inner peace.

Confidence

Are you afraid of failure? Are you afraid of dying? While fear of death has its physiological purposes in self-preservation, it generally impedes growth by blocking constructive risk-taking. Death can come in many varieties. Fear of public speaking feels like a kind of death to many people. Fear of rejection is worse than physical death to others. Some people would rather die than fail their country, their friends, or their values. The most fundamental form of death is loss of the self. Whoever you think you really are – citizen, parent, body, spouse, soul, life – you will tend to defend that self to the death. That is why it is important to learn that you are none of these things. By doing so you do not give up fighting for what is good, harmonious and true; you fight more vigorously for them because you cannot die.

IDL gives voice to perspectives that are not afraid to die in any of these ways. As you practice becoming them your sense of self will first expand, then thin and eventually evaporate, until there is no self to defend and therefore nothing to be afraid of.

All interviewed characters do not share these six characteristics, nor do those who possess some of them necessarily possess them all. There is, however, a tendency for some of your interviewed characters to possess these characteristics to a greater degree than you do, an assertion that you are encouraged to test for yourself. What this implies is that your interviewed characters tend to be more identified with these core life compass qualities than you are. Therefore, if you wish to identify with the agenda of your life compass, you can do worse than identify with those interviewed characters that demonstrate these qualities.

There are several other characteristics of interviewed characters that are important to mention.

Cooperation

About 75% of the time, the interviewed characters in this sample are willing to work together to create a dreamage and to suggest waking changes. In the dream *A Robber is Killed*, both the *two men* (detectives) and their adversary, *Burglar*, are willing to cooperate and form a dreamage, even though they are in fundamental conflict in the dream narrative. It turns out that the *Two Men* really don't want to kill the robber and that *Burglar* really doesn't want to steal, be secretive, or be dishonest. While significant resistance remains to cooperation among some interviewed characters, it is much less than the author expected would be found.

Your interviewed characters are more likely to cooperate with you, on the whole, than are other humans. This is why working first for an internal consensus before attempting social consensus is not only smarter but also easier.

Affect

A statement of preference is a statement of simple like or dislike, which are feelings. Because preferences are statements of feeling as well as perspective, the vast majority of interviewed characters express feelings. Only a few interviewed characters express no preferences. It often happens that interviewed characters in the Dream Sociomatrix Commentary express feelings that were not included in the dream account itself. From these feelings you learn that you feel things you didn't know you felt. You learn that you care about things you've been lying to yourself about. You find that you spend a lot of time and energy pointlessly running from your feelings. Character identification slowly but surely teaches you how to stop such dishonesty.

Depression often involves a sealing off of feelings. Identification with interviewed characters reverses this process. Your waking self begins to identify with perspectives that feel, which is an antidote to depression.

Listening to your wounds

It is important to listen carefully to those interviewed characters that personify various wounded or fixated perspectives. These include abandonment, rejection, death, and failure. If you persist in identifying with the above positive characteristics while ignoring or repressing what wounded perspectives have to say, you will slow down your development. The proper priority is to first focus on defusing whatever pain or hurt is expressed. Then you can more authentically identify with your potentials without simply indulging in sublimation.

Summary

- Because Dream Sociometry is built upon the elicitation of preferences, self-acceptance is its fundamental value and lesson.
- This "self" that you are learning to accept is the entire microcosmic and macrocosmic order.

- Consistently becoming a sociometric star by being most preferred by your interviewed characters requires a consistent willingness to take responsibility for the preferences expressed by interviewed emerging potentials.
- IDL teaches you to accept who you are through carefully listening to both healthy and dysfunctional perspectives, actions, and feelings.
- Every interviewed character personifies some important truth about yourself, whether or not that is its intention. Just because an interviewed character is an isolate or is itself disinterested does not reduce its importance to the group or to the life issues under consideration.
- The more that you identify with characteristics of interviewed perspectives that are of central importance to them, the more you support your evolution into identification with the consciousness of your life compass.

Note

1 "Nightmare" patterns are one type of four basic constellations of elements observed in Dream Sociograms. This is a technical usage, not to be confused with the typical recalled nightmare, that may or may not create this variety of intrasocial group dynamic.

Chapter 16

Structure of the Dream Sociomatrix Commentary

All truth is a species of revelation.

Sir Edward Coke

Collecting and writing the elaborations

As interviewed character preferences are expressed, accompanying explanations, called elaborations, are written down. These are the perspectives, opinions, observations, and feelings of each interviewed character that states preferences. After the first interviewed character on the list, who is always Dream Self, considers its preference toward each element, the second interviewed character states preferences for all elements. These are noted in the Dream Sociomatrix and associated elaborations are written in the Dream Sociomatrix Commentary. This process continues until all interviewed characters have expressed their preferences.

Write elaborations in present tense

Elaborations are always written in the present tense as the character, not you. An example is, "He needs to be locked up or exterminated," not "He needed to be locked up or exterminated." Staying in present tense helps to keep you in the experience clearly and accurately rather than analytically abstracting yourself from it. By expressing all preferences as the appropriate interviewed character would, you maintain role, which is essential. This assures a candidness and honesty that pays great dividends for those who value clarity of their motives and who desire practical help in daily problem solving.

Interviewed characters make their comments in third person, present tense: "Dream Self is OK except when he is trying to take over control of the airplane from me." This language may sound a bit stilted, but is necessary because at the time that you write these words, *you are not the dreamer*. Your assumed perspective is not you. Ideally and theoretically, the two are one, but practically speaking, there is a world of difference between them. From the perspective of interviewed characters, your Dream Self is the "other." Your normal proximate "I" has become just one more distal role you play.

Length

Some interviewed characters will not have much to say. If they don't have preferences to share, leave them alone. Respect their desire not to share. Other interviewed characters will have a lot to say, wanting to comment on each element in the dream. Consequently, there is no firm guideline regarding the length of the Dream Sociomatrix Commentary. Each will spontaneously create itself.

The establishment of a strong identification with each interviewed character is the key to the elicitation of meaningful preferences. It may take some practice to naturally shift into the perspective of several different perspectives. Consequently, once you are in a particular role it is best to learn from it as much as you can before moving on to the next. It is much better to move through the entire dream or life drama a number of times, but each time seeing it through the eyes of a different character, than it is to move through the dream once, addressing each element in turn from the perspective of each.

Underline statements of particular significance

Some statements will jump out at you, even while you are in role. Do not stop to think about them, but do underline them. You will come back and gather these statements in a summary statement later in the process.

Dream consciousness elaborations

If you have chosen to include Dream Consciousness as a chooser in your Dream Sociomatrix, it may express elaborations that explain its purposes for creating the dream. Write them down!

Two follow-up questions

After each interviewed character has expressed its elaborations it is given the opportunity to answer two questions. These are:

What I like most about being in this dream is . . .

and

What I dislike most about being in this dream is . . .

These questions can be thought of as the expression of global preferences by each interviewed character. Each has commented on his or her individual relationships; now it is given the opportunity to comment on its feelings about its participation in the dream as a whole. This tells you what each perspective likes and dislikes most about its participation in the life issues that brought this group together in the first place. It may express its likes and dislikes without necessarily commenting on life issues themselves and those life issues need not be the same as those that are priorities for you.

The two questions asked of Dream Consciousness are different. They are:

What I like most about creating this dream is . . .

and

What I dislike most about creating this dream is . . .

Note whatever responses Dream Consciousness may have to these two questions.

Summary

- Elaborations explain preferences. The statement of preferences provides access to motives that otherwise remain undisclosed.
- When you have a clear understanding of the purposes that motivate your interviewed characters you will usually find that the vast majority of the fear, anger, or sadness that you felt regarding your dream or life drama is needless. This is a powerful experiential permission to approach your life in a more accepting, less reactive way.

Chapter 17

Functions of the Dream
Sociomatrix Commentary

[T]he real friend . . . is, as it were, another self.

Marcus Tullius Cicero

Bringing intention to light

Intention drives preferences and creates perspectives. When intentions are not understood, associated world views, perspectives, and preferences are misperceived. This principle plays itself out in every nightmare. We assume that the intention of a perceived threat is hurtful; we act on that assumption without first gathering information to validate our assumption. In IDL, by creating the Dream Sociomatrix Commentary, you are gathering information about the intentions of perceived threats, antagonists, persecutors, allies and neutral individuals, forces, or objects. When you do so, you are generally confronted with proof that you grossly and routinely misunderstand the intentions of others. The result is the recognition that many of your actions and reactions in both your dreams and your waking life are ignorant or foolish, because they are based on incorrect assumptions about the intentions of others and are therefore self-destructive. At the very least, your misperception of the intentions of others, both awake and dreaming, slows your development; more often, it hinders it.

Through the process of completing the Dream Sociomatrix Commentary, significant feelings, events, and motivations are discovered and more clearly identified. For example, it is not uncommon to find character elaborations that provide information about the dream or life drama that you did not remember but that rings true; you might find you have not just owned a dream car, but stole it five years ago; in the dream *Bicycling Near Hot Springs*, we find that the dreamer's dog, who is running along beside the bicycling dreamer, is "keeping up well," a piece of information about the dream that was not in the dream narrative. In *Lois Clubbing*, Lois, in stating her preferences toward the other dream elements, makes the following comments: "I guess I really don't like clubbing. Why do I do it? It's dishonest, since I'm married. I know he's being dishonest too (Dream Self) when he agrees with me that he thinks it's OK to be out clubbing." While no dislike of clubbing was overtly expressed in the dream, that feeling, with a sense of dishonesty as a motivator, were clearly expressed in the Dream Sociomatrix Commentary.

Anchoring dream events to waking events

Character elaborations build bridges to waking life and thereby anchor the life themes expressed in dream narratives to specific waking events. The dreamer recognized from Lois's comment above that he felt a lot of ambivalence toward the superficial relationship he was pursuing with a woman at the time. He didn't feel that it was honest, even though he was single and not in a relationship with any other woman, but had not clearly recognized that feeling. When you write the elaborations of various monsters, villains and dangerous conditions like fires in Dream Sociomatrix Commentaries, you quickly come to understand two very important, life-changing facts. First, that you routinely scare yourself unnecessarily; second, that things you normally perceive as threats or adversity view themselves as wake-up calls.

Clarifying waking perspectives, feelings, and actions

By creating Dream Sociometric Commentaries, you clarify not only the intentions of others but of yourself as well. Both occur at the same time. One lady had chronic nightmares of a man standing over her while she was sleeping. The elaborations of the man convinced the dreamer that he was an externalization of her life-long habit of constant worry, which she said was a behavior she had learned from her mother. His elaborations also helped her to understand that this man was scaring her because he felt unloved and was angry about abuse he had received as a child. This depth of listening defused both her need to externalize her anger and frighten herself while at the same time reducing her fear of her anger.

Freer expression

The Dream Sociomatrix Commentary allows you to objectively state awarenesses about yourself that you might not otherwise acknowledge. In the dream, *My Counterfeit Mother*, anger that the dreamer would normally not recognize is expressed. The *Large Old House* says, "These people (a woman and man) don't belong in me. They're freeloaders and selfish." The *Woman* in the dream is at least as candid: "Those little brats (two children) had better keep their mouths shut." Whether such perspectives are valid or moral is a completely different issue. Recognizing that such feelings are honest expressions of some aspect of ourselves is an important first step to addressing their cause.

Increased ownership/responsibility

You recognize feelings, actions, and values that you did not even realize that you possessed when you give voice to other perspectives as Dream Sociomatrix elaborations. You are faced with important opportunities for self-acceptance when you read the elaborations of interviewed characters, recognizing them as your own. In the dream *Reconsidering Getting a Car*, the *Old Car* says, "Look, I'm sorry I didn't have good brakes. Don't blame me. Blame my designers." To the extent that the dreamer created this experience, albeit out of his awareness, the car is an aspect of himself. *He* is the designer and is faced with accepting responsibility for not placing proper controls on his actions. In this regard, the Dream Sociogram Commentary becomes a process of accepting responsibility for perspectives, feelings and actions that have previously run your life outside your waking awareness. In this instance, the car recommended replacement with a "better model" – improved control over impulses.

Increased understanding of dreams

When you review the elaborations of an interviewed character, you gain understanding as to why it thinks it is in your dream, why it does what it does, and why it feels what it feels. The character reveals its intentions and meanings to you without recourse to symbols, dream dictionaries, interpreters, or pre-supposition. For example, in the dream *Neighborhood Religion*, the *Church* says, referring to Dream Self, "He shouldn't live in me. It makes me look too gaudy, too much like a home instead of a religious institution. I do not belong in a residential neighborhood or to be treated like a residence." This was an important statement for the dreamer, who had assumed that he was improving his daily life by adding sacred religious elements to it. This elaboration by another interviewed perspective caused him to consider that perhaps he was merely secularizing the sacred rather than making sacred the secular. Armed with the input of various perspectives, you are free to arrive at your *own* conclusion about what the dream "means" or does not "mean." This provides you with important knowledge that will help you to understand dreams and dreaming from a broader, more adequate perspective.

New awareness of sources of inner conflict

As you listen to the comments of interviewed perspectives in the elaborations of the Dream Sociomatrix Commentary, you begin to see how you unnecessarily wage war upon yourself. In the dream *Vicious Horses*, *Three Horses* say, "He (Dream Self) is on our territory. We don't trust him. He better leave us alone or we'll get him. We're tough and independent. We'll show him. Oh, we don't really want to kill him, just teach him a good lesson – get him to respect us." The *Farm* in the same dream then comments, "I would prefer to do without all this fear and meanness disturbing my tranquility. Those horses would leave him alone if he wasn't afraid and wasn't trying to be sneaky." Clearly, the dreamer is disregarding the needs of perspectives personified by these horses, making them angry. *Farm* states that the dreamer is creating this inner reaction by his fear and dishonesty. It became clear to the dreamer from all this that he was afraid of failing at his new job and lying to himself about it.

Ideas for waking application

By enhancing your awareness of yourself, the Dream Sociomatrix Commentary provides an essential ingredient for behavioral change. *Lois Clubbing* led to a defining of those actions that seemed artificial or dishonest in the dreamer's dating relationships and the discussing of those issues with his partner. *My Counterfeit Mother* helped the dreamer to recognize his anger at some lazy, dishonest habits and to confront them more directly. *Neighborhood Religion* caused the dreamer to put less emphasis on acting religious and more on fully benefiting from meditation.

Increased communication with sources of support and direction

As you listen to the elaborations in the Dream Sociomatrix Commentary you strengthen your contact with powerful perspectives that often have clearer, healthier intentions than you do. You now have new allies that you can ask for assistance in problem solving, that are always there and thereby allow you to move beyond loneliness or feelings of separation. By taking on such perspectives at pivotal moments you can reprogram your awareness for enhanced physical and mental health, work satisfaction, and improved interpersonal relationships. In the dream *Extraterrestrials Descend*, the dreamer receives information that turns out to be precognitive. The elaborations of the Dream Sociomatrix Commentary indicated that the dream had to do with a move to Phoenix, Arizona, and was instrumental in making the critical contact that resulted in a work opportunity opening up there.

Insight into self-destructive choices

Perhaps most importantly, you learn when, why, and how you have chosen destruction and failure instead of growth and success. You learn how to choose integration in your daily activities, thoughts, and relationships. In the dream *Fun with Snakes*, the *Snakes* say, "I wish he'd (Dream Self) leave me alone. He's harassing us. We're quality stuff and don't hurt anyone. We wrap around his finger for security. Then he pulls our security out from under us. No wonder we get angry!" As the elaborations of the interviewed characters proceeded, it became clear to the dreamer that he was sometimes having sex just to please his partner, "wrapping her around his finger" so to speak. This was causing friction between them. He realized he needed to take his partner and his sexual expression more seriously.

Here is an example of a Dream Sociomatrix Commentary. It is from *Ken Wilber Dies:*

Dream Self: I like myself a lot because I respect the integrity of my life and my efforts to live in balance and teach others to do so. I love Ken Wilber because I see him doing the same and being much more successful at it than I am. I like his girlfriend because she is meaningful to him; I really don't know much about her except the little I've read about her in *One Taste*. I have no feelings one way or the other about the cars. He is probably driving and it's probably a jeep. The other car seems to be a new model in good shape as well. I hate that there is a head-on crash, that they are killed and that I am very upset. I want to dislike the other driver a lot and blame him for the crash, but I don't know if that is accurate or not. What I like most about being in this dream is nothing. I feel like I'm not in it, but a spectator who gets the news. What I dislike most about being in this dream is the sense of tragedy and loss that I feel.

Ken Wilber: I love Joseph for his dedication and out of my desire that he, as well as many others, carry on my work, now that I can't. I love myself because I have lived my life in a way that has reflected my ideals to the best of my ability. I love my girlfriend very much and really hate that she died too. I like my car and feel terrible that it's now destroyed. The second car I have no feelings about. I hate the needless waste of this head-on collision. It was unnecessary and entirely avoidable. I hate it that I have to die unnecessarily and for no good purpose. I like a lot that Joseph is very upset. He should be. I dislike the other driver because he caused this wreck! What I like most about being in this dream is nothing! What I dislike most about being in this dream is getting killed for no good reason or purpose. It's so futile!

Girlfriend: I really appreciate Joseph's concern. I love Ken very much! I like myself a lot and feel really bad that I am dead. It feels so needless and meaningless. I don't like that other car a lot because it killed us, which I hate. I like a lot that Joseph is very upset; he should be! The other driver was thoughtless. His negligence not only ended his life but ours too! What I like most about being in this dream is being recalled so that I can now express my anger about being killed needlessly! What I dislike most about being in this dream is losing Ken and losing my life, all out of thoughtless, brain dead, mindless, sleepwalking through life on the part of the other driver. He swerved in front of us!

Car:	I feel pretty much like everybody else so far, except that I like myself a lot and really hate that I had a head on crash. I feel that I didn't do my job and let Ken and his girlfriend down, although I can't see how I could have done anything differently. I hate the other driver! What I like most about being in this dream is having a chance to express how much I hate this!! What I dislike most about being in this dream is playing the victim. I know I'm not really dead, because I'm talking right now, but I don't have the same physical reality that I would have if I had continued to live in that dream!
Second Car:	I don't know any of these people but I feel terrible that I killed them! I guess they were pretty special and now they're gone! I am pretty upset too because I was alive, doing my job and now I'm gone and I can't! My driver was thoughtless and inconsiderate. I don't like him at all! What I like most about being in this dream is that I have the opportunity to express myself by being recalled and listened to. What I dislike most about being in this dream is that I am the instrument by which insensitivity and injustice occurs.
Other Driver:	I pretty much agree with everyone else. I WAS to blame! I was thoughtless, insensitive and careless. I hate it that I killed these people and myself. Dream Self has every right to be upset with me! I am upset with myself very much! I hate myself for what I did! What I like most about being in this dream is nothing. What I dislike most about being in this dream is being responsible for all this needless tragedy!
Dream Consciousness:	I love all these characters that I created. I am sorry that they are so upset! It's really not necessary! What I want them to do is see beyond their expectations and be thankful in all circumstances, even those that seem unfair and unjust. What I like most about creating this dream is demonstrating how even great tragedy can be seen in a broader context devoid of drama. What I dislike most about creating this dream is that I had to go to these lengths to get Joseph's attention to teach him this truth. If he would just accept it and practice it, I wouldn't have to scare him to get his attention!

What surprises me about what I've heard is

Obviously, the above comments add a great deal of interpretation, from multiple perspectives, to the perspective of the dreamer when he wrote the dream narrative and his initial associations to the dream. His awareness had been broad-ened. By becoming all these different perspectives, he has broadened and thinned his sense of self. He has given himself an experience in multi-perspectivalism, which is a fundamental characteristic of the transpersonal because it involves the deconstruction of the self and of psychological geocentrism. As you prac-tice deep listening to your interviewed characters, you will be struck by the implications of this or that elaboration. This section, "What surprises me about what I've heard is," allows you to journal those awarenesses in one place as they come to you. Just skip down to this section, and jot down whatever surprises you about what you've heard this or that interviewed character say. Then return to eliciting preferences and writing elaborations in the Dream Sociomatrix Commentary.

Here is an example of "What surprises me about what I've heard is" from *Ken Wilber Dies:*

What surprises me about what I've heard is . . . I notice that I care about another character more strongly than I do about myself. I also notice that I have very strong negative preferences, which doesn't feel particularly enlightened! It is curious to me that I have no concern for the driver of the other car. I don't even include him as a character, although I should! I will go back and add him in . . .

Ken Wilber appears to more or less be a surrogate because his preferences are pretty much the same as mine. The exception is that he likes a lot that I am very upset, which makes sense, from his perspective, but the preference ends up being opposite that of Dream Self. He provides new information – that the crash was indeed an accident and that it was caused by the other driver.

The girlfriend is also a surrogate of the dreamer because her preferences are very similar, but even a bit harder, more polarized because she dislikes the second car, where Dream Self does not. I don't think I've ever had a character say that what it liked most about being in a dream was "being recalled" so that the character could express its feelings! She states that the other driver swerved in front of them.

This reminds me of some thoughts that I had yesterday or the day before as I was driving. I was thinking about teaching (my daughter) Kira how to drive (she's thirteen) and about how I wanted to teach her to pray for other drivers, about how any of them at any time could swerve in front of her or pull out in front of her, about how we drive taking for granted that other drivers are going to do what they need to do to keep us safe, but in fact our lives are always in the hands of oncoming drivers and any one of them could change the course of our lives forever. So I started praying for the other drivers and thought about how doing so changes the consciousness of the cells of my body, especially the water, which makes up 90+ % of my body. I imagined those cells transformed into perfect patterns of thankfulness and appreciation.

The car is ambivalent toward itself, liking itself but disliking itself for "letting Ken and his girlfriend down."

The remarks of the second car remind me of my recent loss of my father and before that, my mother. They were pretty special and now they're gone. I am surprised that the second car, which is blamed in part for the wreck, is also angry and blaming its driver, because it is dead too!

The awareness of all these characters that they are not "really" dead because they still can express their feelings contradicts their anger at having their paths disrupted. Do they have reason to be really upset or not? Are they dead or not? It would seem that they are not and that therefore they are all overreacting at the fact that their path has been interrupted and therefore their live path has not lived up to their expectations. It sounds like the crash isn't the problem, but their expectations that the crash was unfair is the problem!

Other Driver is a part of myself that thinks it is itself bad because it does stupid, tragic, thoughtless things. Because it makes bad choices, it punishes itself. The thought that comes to my mind is "How much do I need to beat up on myself when I kill the best parts of myself? How long do I need to blame myself or stay on a guilt trip when I slip up and destroy the best parts of myself? Is it really helpful? Does it really change anything?" I also realize that in so doing I am not distinguishing between who I am and what I do. I am not "loving the actor but hating the action." After all, this IS a dream! We, Dream Self and the various characters in the dream, could all learn from our experience, laugh about the intensity of our feelings and get on with our lives.

I need to practice being thankful in all situations, just as I was reminding myself and practicing as I was driving the other day. This dream came to strongly reinforce that practice and that perspective. I need not waste time beating myself up when I screw up!

Such conclusions reflect the practical applications that can result from putting both dream and life dramas in perspective. Notice that Dream Sociometry merges dream and life dramas. From the perspective of life, there is no difference, because each is the mirror of the other and by awakening within one you awaken within the other.

The other commentaries

Your work completing your Dream Sociomatrix and the Dream Sociomatrix Commentary will reflect your life issues at the time you work on the dream and not necessarily the issues that generated the dream itself. You will find that working on one dream a week or one every other week will generate enough "homework" to keep you out of any trouble you might otherwise find the time to get into. Just as it is not necessary to take your blood pressure every day, it is not necessary to evaluate a new intrasocial group every day in order to receive the feedback you need to improve your psychological, physical, interpersonal, and transpersonal health. Completing a Dream Sociomatrix occasionally, just as you occasionally go to the doctor for a physical and have your blood taken, is a necessary and sufficient prevention. You do not have to become a dream researcher or make creation of Dream Sociomatrices a regular, ongoing part of your integral life practice in order to gain great and lasting benefit from it.

In addition to the Dream Sociometric Commentary, the Dream Commentary and Waking Commentaries help you apply the recommendations of your interviewed characters in your life. These will be covered in subsequent chapters.

When to complete the Dream Sociogram

The Dream Sociogram is an educational and research tool that provides a visual picture of the relationships among the preferences expressed by a particular group of dream or life drama perspectives.

As an educational tool it can be used with students to help them understand and resolve internal conflicts while accessing and strengthening their intrasocial support system. As a research tool the Dream Sociogram clarifies types of intrasocial groups that are naturally formed by patterns of preference, discloses their interactions as well as the implications of those relationships for both health and transformation. While the Dream Sociogram does not have to be constructed at the same time the Dream Sociomatrix and Dream Sociomatrix Commentary are created, a better continuity and understanding are provided if these are done together. If a choice is to be made, it is preferable to proceed to the Dream Commentary, Dreamage, Waking Commentary, and Action Plan and return to the Dream Sociogram later, because the various commentaries provide important interpretive background that informs how you view and understand a Dream Sociogram.

Summary

- Statements by interviewed characters in the Dream Sociomatrix Commentary provide additional important information about dreams and life dramas, correct your misperceptions, clarify and contribute feelings, reveal perspectives and feelings you hold but that you were unaware of, and give birth to new intentions, perspectives, and possibilities that heal, balance, and transform your life.
- It is common for us to avoid responsibility because of the shame and guilt that often accompanies our failure to meet our responsibilities. IDL encourages ownership of our responsibilities but within the context of a broader self-acceptance. This neutralizes the shame and guilt which serve as forms of self-persecution that keep us trapped in the Drama Triangle.
- The various commentaries throw light on our motivations while disclosing useful approaches to the resolution of long-standing internal conflicts.

Chapter 18

Overview of commentary construction and creation of the Action Plan

---

The action commentaries

It's better to aim at the moon and miss than to aim at a skunk and hit it.

The goal of the Dream Commentary, Dreamage, Waking Commentary, Identification Commentary, Reading Back "I" Statements, Action Plan, Dream Sociogram Commentary, Group Dynamics Commentary, and Group Feedback Commentary is to anchor your interviews in your daily life.

What do your interviewed characters aspire to? There are four basic questions that can be asked of dreams and life dramas, each of which corresponds to a different holon quadrant:

1) What is the perspective or world view of this dream or life drama?

   (The interior collective quadrant of meanings, culture and values.)

2) What does the overall level of development represented by this dream or life drama?

   (The interior individual quadrant of consciousness, thoughts, and feelings.)

3) How does this dream or life drama affect my relationship with others?

   (The exterior collective quadrant of relationships and society.)

4) What do I want to do with this dream or life drama?

   (The exterior individual quadrant of behavior.)

The different commentaries focus on addressing these different questions in different ways.

The *Dream Summary Commentary* asks each interviewed character to state,

My strengths are . . .
My weaknesses or limitations are . . .

The aspects of this dreamer that I most closely personify are . . .
The reason why I am in this dream is . . .
(Dream Consciousness:) The reason why I created this dream is . . . This dream (or
life drama) group came together to . . .

Strengths and limitations could be in behavior, development, values, or relationships, indicating in which quadrants each character perceives its strengths and
in which its limitations.

Creating the *Dreamage* is a behavioral recommendation – repeating the
changed dream, if one can be created – before sleep as an incubated pre-sleep
suggestion. It is designed to generate changes in dream consciousness (internal
individual quadrant) and values/perspectives, both while dreaming and awake
(internal collective quadrant.

The Waking Commentary focuses on changes in all four quadrants by asking,
If I were this dreamer and lived his waking life for her, how would I live it differently?
Would I handle her three life issues differently? If so, how? Recommendations may
involve changes in behavior, perspective, thinking and feeling, and interactions
with others.

The *Identification Commentary* focuses on evolution of the interior collective quadrant by identifying times and circumstances in which it would
be helpful for the dreamer to become this or that emerging potential and
respond as it would.

Reading back "I" Statements is a way to make changes in the internal collective quadrant by taking responsibility for who you are and the reality you
have created.

The *Action Plan* emphasizes behavioral change in the individual and collective
exterior quadrants of the human holon. Many people hate setting goals because
they experience them as pressure, and they are already self-critical. They already
feel that they are failing to live up to their expectations; why should they make
themselves feel worse by taking on even more goals and responsibilities? The
result of this false reasoning is that we either do not set goals or never learn
how to set realistic ones. The result is our lives become a product of the goals
of others; we spend our lives fulfilling the dreams of those who know how to
set and pursue attainable goals. Not setting realistic goals or refusing to work
toward them daily is to say, "I like being a victim." "I want to stay powerless so
I have reason to whine and blame others for my own immaturity."

IDL understands the strong, natural resistances to goal setting and attainment
that is shared by all of us. It addresses these concerns by showing you how to
set goals that matter to *you*, not to others and how to make them small and
simple enough so that your work toward them is satisfying and rewarding rather
than aversive and frustrating. The following commentaries are designed to help
you apply what you have learned from the Dream Sociomatrix and the Dream
Sociomatrix Commentary.

The *Sociogram Commentary* provide your interpretations of the relationships among the choosers and chosen in the Dream Sociomatrix. This involves an expansion of the interior collective quadrant.

The *Group Dynamics Commentary* provide your interpretations of the relationships among the choosers and chosen in the Dream Sociomatrix. This involves an expansion of the interior collective quadrant.

Group Feedback Commentary provides interpretations of the relationships among the choosers and chosen in the Dream Sociomatrix by the various interviewed characters themselves. This involves an expansion of the interior collective quadrant.

Summary

- The various commentaries focus on making your dream experience a living and vital part of your waking life.
- Your goal is to deeply listen to those emerging potentials that need healing and those emerging potentials that provide enlightenment and support your development.
- The commentaries provide a map for aligning your waking priorities with those of your life compass, in the theory that attunement to the agenda of your life compass amplifies your ability to express life's agenda in your world.

Chapter 19

The Dream Summary Commentary

To understand the heart and mind of a person, look not at what he has already achieved, but at what he aspires to.

Kahlil Gibran

Each interviewed perspective answers the following five statements in what is called the Dream Summary Commentary:

> *My strengths are . . .*
> *My weaknesses or limitations are . . .*
> *The aspects of this dreamer that I most closely personify are . . .*
> *The reason why I am in this dream or life drama is . . .*
> *(Dream Consciousness:) The reason why I created this dream or life drama is . . .*
> *This dream (or life drama) group came together to . . .*

The Dream Summary Commentary gives your interviewed characters the opportunity to answer these questions from their perspective. This takes much of the guesswork, not to mention the pontificating, out of dreamwork. It also makes dream interpretation a cooperative effort with deference to your intra-social community.

The first statement, "*My strengths are*," clarifies those attributes of the interviewed character that it considers to be particularly noteworthy. This reveals strengths that you may or may not have recognized. In either case, this information reveals resources represented by this character. It provides each character with an opportunity to elaborate on its strong points. If it has been discounted or rejected by the dreamer, an awareness of its strengths is essentially an awareness by the dreamer of his or her disowned strengths. For example, a hospital says "I don't have any fear of abandonment. I'm well adjusted. I don't have any of your fears. I don't fear my existence being terminated." This was very unlike the dreamer, who had both fears of abandonment and fears of death.

The second statement, "*My weaknesses or limitations are*," identifies those attributes of the interviewed character that it considers to be challenges or limitations, whether you do or not. It provides information about how the dreamer is blocking their own development. Of course, those things that are perceived as limitations are often strengths when rightly understood, just as nightmare persecutors are often sources of important awakening when we take the time to listen to them.

The third statement, "*The aspects of this dreamer that I most closely personify are,*" provides the character with an opportunity to identify those aspects of the dreamer that it most clearly represents. This statement goes a long way toward clearing up any lingering theoretical doubts about whether or not an interviewed character is indeed an aspect of the dreamer. This question implies that the interviewed character does, in fact, personify some aspect of you. Even if an interviewed character is Jesus or a deceased relative it will still personify one or more aspects of you. This is because we inherently project meaning onto all experience and all others. You own your projections and consider those meanings and values each interviewed character chooses as most significant. For example, if you have a dream visitation by your deceased grandmother, was it really her? IDL says this is the wrong question to ask because there is no definitive way to answer it. Instead it asks, "If grandmother were an aspect of me, what parts would she personify?" "If grandmother were indeed herself, an external reality that is coming to me in this experience, so what?" "What conclusions do I draw from the belief that she is real?" Does it mean that something or someone exists that I am not?" "If everything and everybody is really a part of me, how is that not solipsism?"

This question also provides each interviewed character with an opportunity to interpret its own significance in relationship to the waking life of the dreamer. How relevant and important is that? Once you have had some experience with this level of interpretive input, you will most likely find that while the contributions of other sources, such as psychics and books on dream interpretation, can provide new depths and textures of meaning, they can never take the place of the contributions of your interviewed emerging potentials.

You provide your interviewed characters with the opportunity to interpret the meaning of their own experience. While their responses do not necessarily preempt interpretive comments from books, therapists, or other dreamworkers, they take priority. This is because the feedback of your interviewed characters about themselves is assumed to be more informed than others.

You will find that your interviewed characters are not bashful about telling you those perspectives that they most closely personify. Here are some examples from a variety of interviewed characters:

School bus: I most closely personify confusion, overwhelm.

Baby: I personify the dreamer's deepest, true self. I am her true self that's ready to be nurtured in the world and by herself too. My strengths are goal vision and trusting a heck of a lot more. I'm really trusting. At this point I can see her as more trusting than any other time in her life.

Hawk: I personify the awakening that she has the same kind of eye-sight that I do. She can see underneath the surface of things.

River: I personify how the dreamer has a still, slow, quiet personality but that she can still be very deep and powerful. She is flow-ing all right. She is going in the right direction.

White Bathroom: I personify her emotions. She was not allowed to express her emotions as a child. It felt stark. All the time she was flooded with emotions.

The fourth statement, "*The reason why I am in this dream is,*" provides each inter-viewed character with the opportunity to interpret its significance within your life. This question is meant to address any individual issues that the character has which are being expressed through its participation in the dream. It may address any or all of the four quadrants. It provides an opportunity for the interviewed character to explain its intent or purpose, which is an internal individual quad-rant concern. In addition, the question certainly speaks to meaning and value issues of the internal collective quadrant. The reasons why an interviewed char-acter is in a dream often relate to both the dreamer's waking behavior (indi-vidual external quadrant) and their relationship with others, both other aspects of themselves with whom they may be in conflict and other individuals. This question also provides a window on the life issues that concern the interviewed character, which may be quite different from those of the dreamer.

Here are examples of answers to this question:

Lois: I most closely personify the insecure, easily threatened part of the dreamer, a part that is in need of approval. The reason why I am in this dream is to point out that I am still here, but latent. I can get threatened easily and the reason why is because I am insecure and I need approval.

We can see from this comment that this character has a purpose of calling its continued existence to the attention of the dreamer, who had tended to assume it was a perspective that was no longer an issue. Insecurity and approval are personal emotional reactions. As behaviors, they are aspects of the dreamer's individual external quadrant. As reactions to the perceived intentions and actions of others, they indicate an important relationship with the external collective quadrant.

Here is another interviewed character from the same dream:

Couch: I most closely personify both casual comfort and meditation. You meditate on a couch like me every morning. The rea-son why I am in this dream is to emphasize that the context of your meditation is what was missing before and what is present now that is bringing a necessary, but previously dead, part of yourself back to life.

In this dream, the dreamer's father, who had died over a year previously, showed up at the door. The couch indicates that the cultivation of a meditative consciousness, an individual interior issue, is a priority for it. It also indicates that it supports meditation, an individual exterior behavior.

The reason why I created this dream is

Dream Consciousness answers this question in a slightly different form: *The reason why I created this dream is.*

Here is Dream Consciousness' response to these three concerns in the above dream:

Dream consciousness: I most closely personify transcendent witnessing that watches your life drama, both conscious and unconscious, with equanimity and acceptance. The reason why I created this dream is to provide a metaphorical expression of the relationship between the meditation you are doing and the healing of pretty deeply buried issues of inadequacy, insecurity and the need of the approval of others. This intrasocial group came together to speed that process through reducing and hopefully eliminating your waking resistance to its surfacing and to hopefully motivate you to support and encourage this healing process. You do so when you meditate and when you listen to your interviewed characters as you are now doing.

Your Dream Consciousness will express what it personifies in its own words. Don't assume that this expression is correct or right or that it should serve as a model. You will do much better if you let your Dream Consciousness be and say whatever it spontaneously feels.

The fifth statement, "*This dream (or life drama) group came together to*," provides your choosing perspectives with an opportunity to interpret the dream as a whole. Notice that the wording does not bias the interpretation toward what relevance it may have for the dreamer and his or her concerns. The intrasocial group may have an agenda that is only indirectly related to your waking life issues. It is important to remain open to this possibility, because you can thereby learn a great deal about what you are ignoring, repressing, or simply have not recognized.

When a number of interviewed characters answer this question you begin to get a sense that you know why you had the dream or life drama, at least from the points of view of an assortment of invested perspectives. When these explanations are correlated with the answer to this statement provided by Dream Consciousness, most dreamers feel that they have a much clearer sense of why they had the dream or are experiencing a particular life drama.

Here are two examples of responses to this question. They are continuations of the answers provided by Lois and Couch above.

Lois: This intrasocial group came together to help you get out of the way and let there be a healing of the part of yourself that is like me by a surfacing of that part of yourself which is like your father. That part loves me unconditionally and therefore is not critical or threatening toward me.

Couch: This intrasocial group came together to explain how your meditation is resurrecting joyful and non-judgmental perspectives.

These were aspects of the dream that felt right to the dreamer but had not been anticipated by the original dream. Out of this came not only understanding and insight but increased motivation for mediation and a way to avoid marital friction. The part of the dreamer that was like his father could be brought to the forefront to deal with his wife when she was like Lois, thereby avoiding personalization and overreaction by the dreamer to his wife.

After the choosing interviewed characters are given the opportunity to respond to these three issues, you may want to ask Dream Consciousness to respond as well.

Here is the Dream Summary Commentary for *Ken Wilber Dies:*[1]

Ken Wilber: I most closely personify the parts of Joseph that he admires and respects the most, the parts that are dedicated to service but which balance it with a healthy dedication to balancing body, mind and life in his own life. The reason why I am in this dream is to help him let go of his expectations that he grow into me, to feel OK about who he is right now and where he is right now. Life is always going to be an interrupted journey. This intrasocial group came together to teach moment to moment non-attachment, thankfulness and appreciation.

Girlfriend: I most closely personify the more emotionally attached, caring part of Joseph. I hate not being able to be supportive, because that's how I justify my existence! The reason why I am in this dream is to let go of the need to do that. This intrasocial group came together to help Joseph understand, through working through it, that life goes on, even when it doesn't live up to his expectations. Therefore, he needs to drop his unrealistic expectations and his guilt when he doesn't live up to them.

Car: I most closely personify Joseph's body. The reason why I am in this dream is to help him let go of his fear of physical death so that he can live more courageously as he grows older. This intrasocial group came together to teach love in all circumstances, even the most painful ones.

Second Car: I most closely personify the parts of your physical life that are self- destructive and end up even destroying itself, such as bad eating habits or out-of-control genes that cause your body to break down regardless of what you do. The reason why I am in this dream is to help you to learn compassion toward your own self-destruction. This intrasocial group came together to help you gain objectivity toward the drama of your fears, your expectations and your self-blame.

Other Driver: I most closely personify the part of you that makes stupid choices out of lack of discernment or unawareness. The reason why I am in this dream is to get you to accept that this is a natural part of yourself and that while you may succeed in reducing it somewhat, it will always be there, so you might as well develop some compassion toward it! This intrasocial group came together to get you to let go of your sense of unfairness or injustice, particularly regarding your relationship with the mother of your daughter.

Dream Consciousness: I most closely personify the part of you that loves you enough to put you through pain in order to help you wake up. The reason why I created this dream is to help you let go of your expectations and learn to watch yourself go by. This intrasocial group came together to cultivate your identification with the witness.

Summary

- The overall level of development indicated by a dream or life drama is determined not by the highest or lowest consciousness expressed within it but as an average of all participants. The consciousness of each individual interviewed character is determined by its preferences and its elaborations, as well as by self and peer assessments of it.
- Dream meanings are best determined by interviewed characters themselves. After all, it is *their* dream or life drama.
- Before taking action based on what you think your dream is about, it is wise to consult other, equally invested perspectives.
- Before you conclude that a dream is nonsense or contains the New Revelation for Mankind it is wise to consult other, equally invested perspectives.
- The questions in the Dream Summary Commentary are designed to clarify all four of these aspects of the holon of your life.

Note

1 Underlining indicates particularly cogent statements that are written as "I" statements in the associated commentary below.

Chapter 20

Constructing the Dreamage

The greatest happiness of the greatest number is the foundation of morals and legislation.
Jeremy Bentham

Purpose of the Dreamage

The Dreamage (dream + image) is a dream rewritten to reflect the stated preferences of your interviewed characters. It reflects collective character opinion arrived at through a consensual or democratic process . . . *a degree of agreement regarding goals, norms, rules and other aspects of the group.*[1] Such cohesiveness gives rise to "solidarity," which is *the stabilized mutual responsibility of each toward the other to regard himself as part of the other, as the sharer of a common fate and as a person who is under obligation to cooperate with the other in the satisfaction of the other's individual needs as if they were one's own.*[2] Reorganization of a dream or life drama to have maximum positive impact can never be the expression of your preferences to the exclusion of those of other perspectives, because such a reorganization will respect and include the preferences of as broad a collective of preferences as possible.[3] A dreamage never reflects the will of the dreamer at the expense of any group member. The consent and endorsement of all characters interviewed is required before a restructured dream qualifies to be called a dreamage.

Why create a dreamage?

Eugene Ionesco has said, "Fantasy is revealing; it is a method of cognition. Everything that is imagined is true, nothing is true if it is not imagined." We change the truth of our lives while we sleep. We can participate in this process by recognizing that our dreams are a form of feedback that can be integrated for maximum positive impact and then used as a potent form of input into the sleep problem solving process. This is a fundamental rationale for the construction of a dreamage. The basic purpose of the Dream Commentary question is to encourage the development of an accepting, cooperative approach among *all* invested aspects of self. Because dreamages are metaphorical statements of the elimination of internal conflict regarding those life issues that gave rise to the dream or life drama, they amplify contact with transpersonal or normative awareness, which increases access to objectivity, wisdom, love, and creativity.

Your dreamage acts as a suggestion, in the organic language of your body and mind, that there is now being experienced an ideal solution to the life issues expressed in your dream. The dreamage puts in motion alternative, integrative approaches to the resolution of those issues of interest to the intrasocial group. It can be thought of as a type of medicine designed for you and you alone that works to heal conflicting internal relationships, focusing your life toward growth. It does so by addressing the needs of previously opposed or divisive interests, perspectives, and life patterns and transforming them into synergistic and negentropic processes.

A dreamage may be visualized prior to sleep in order to support integrative, life compass-based perspectives in your dreams. Dreamages reduce dream stress by introducing powerful suggestions for harmonious interactions among your various interviewed characters. These in turn subtly alter your waking life. In addition, dreamages may be used as visual affirmations during waking hours to support integration and conflict resolution.

Why not simply construct a positive revision of a dream and work with it instead of going through the process of asking your interviewed characters to create a dreamage? You can answer this question for yourself. Choose a dream with some conflict in it for which you plan to complete a Dream Sociomatrix. Before beginning, write down your concept of what the dreamage will be. Now, create the Dream Sociomatrix Commentary and the Dream Commentary. Now, let your interviewed characters submit their proposals for a dreamage. Can they agree to create a dreamage? If they do, how closely does theirs resemble yours? How are they different? Sometimes you will be close, but sometimes you will not, because you are guessing at what integration would look like for other perspectives. Just as a part is hardly in a position to comprehend the whole, so your waking identity does not always understand or represent your broader needs. If it did, you would have a much clearer perception of your problems and their solutions. You would find yourself much less frequently in conflict with yourself.

Your waking version of integration, as expressed in such a pseudo-dreamage, is unlikely to be as constructive as that of the dreamage itself. This is because it is unlikely to reflect the desires of *all* invested perspectives present among interviewed characters, as the dreamage does. It is unlikely to speak as clearly and powerfully to the autonomic nervous system as does a dreamage because it will not have been created in the same spontaneous way that the dream was.[4] While it is relatively easy for two countries to unilaterally arm themselves and attack each other, it is another thing entirely for those countries to interdependently disarm and make peace. Any of us can unilaterally bring our will to bear on some life problem; it is another matter entirely to make appropriate changes as an equal, cooperative *partner* with other invested perspectives. Our failure to appreciate this distinction is a fundamental way we create unhappiness and pain in our lives. We habitually act unilaterally without taking the needs of broader, collective perspectives into account.

Construction of the dreamage supports intrasocial group integration by increasing consensus and cohesion. Intrinsic, dream-based imagery has a particular cogency and impact on consciousness. It affects you in an organic way that imagery created for you by others does not. It metaphorically depicts spontaneously derived, collective alternatives to conflict that transcend your waking world view and preferences. It is therefore likely to be integrative. The metaphorical nature of your interviewed emerging potentials speaks uniquely to you. Through the attainment of goals desired by both Dream Self and a consensus of interviewed characters, the dreamage works to harmonize the needs of your waking identity with the perspectives, values, and agenda of your life compass. Schizmogenetic[5] divisions that are routinely taken for granted and considered "normal," between intrasocial perspectives and that of your waking identity, are transcended. No longer does your right hand not know what the left one is doing.

Visualizations created by a teacher or therapist or by your waking self can be powerfully transformative. IDL does not suggest that you choose use of dreamages over other types of visualization, but rather that you broaden your repertoire to include both.

Some dreams will be their own dreamage

Those intrasocial groups whose patterns of preferences are *synthesis*, that is, consistently positive, will generally serve as their own dreamage. In such a case, choosers will recommend no changes be made when asked the Dream Commentary question. They will usually want to keep the dream just as it is. Such a group is inherently constructive and personifies a high level of internal acceptance regarding the issues that generated the intrasocial group in the first place. It is beneficial to work with this sort of dream as a dreamage, because doing so reinforces innate patterns of harmonious functioning in body, mind and life. Examples of this type of dream include most synthesis patterns.[6]

While it is possible that your life dramas will serve as their own dreamage, this is unlikely. Even in the unlikely case that all interviewed perspectives agree that the life situation should stay the way it is, Dream Self is likely to be the holdout. However, it is conceivable that the process of listening to the various commentaries will convince Dream Self to change his or her mind regarding the toxicity of the life drama. In such a case, a life drama could indeed become its own dreamage.

When consensus is not feasible

In some intrasocial groups, consent will not be so easily won. What happens if one character refuses to join a consensus? Let's say the *Other Driver* in *Ken Wilber*

Dies refuses to do anything but blame himself for causing the wreck. Consider destructive or persecuting interviewed characters as ignored or rejected perspectives that have become "louder" in their words or actions in order to grab attention and motivate change. Instead of being defensive, think, "This group member personifies a disenfranchised or impulsive perspective.[7] It is so needy that it is lashing out like some wounded animal. What can I do to relieve its pain, to respect and respond to its plight?" Socially, this reasoning can sound like criminal coddling by "bleeding heart liberals" that prepersonal and early personal perspectives love to bash. However, in the intrasocial universe other approaches do not seem to work so well. This is because to condemn or force an intrasocial group member is to condemn or force *yourself*, which generally only creates more resistance. This is an example of how IDL tends to infuse higher personal and transpersonal perspectives into prepersonal and personal consciousness.

All parties must feel comfortable with the dreamage

> *But to manipulate men, to propel them towards goals which you – the social reformers – see, but they may not, is to deny their human essence, to treat them as objects without wills of their own and therefore to degrade them.*
>
> Sir Isaiah Berlin

The implied discounting of invested perspectives through exclusion is an excellent reason why interviewed characters are to be consulted before dreams are restructured to act as suggestions for self-change. Parts of you resist change and for their own good reasons. You need to listen to that resistance instead of blithely assuming that you know what is best for others. You can easily get in touch with perspectives that are immature, impulsive, selfish, and addicted to drama, which enjoy superiority within their own groups and resent interference, others who believe it is appropriate to be treated as less than equal, and others still who have grown comfortable in the stability bondage offers. Help those who seek it, learn from those who know more than you do, and respect the resistance or silence of the rest.

Do not attempt to create a dreamage that is not acceptable *all* involved interviewed characters. On rare occasions, mentioned above, a dreamage can be constructed without the participation of resistive interviewed characters, but only if they decide not to block it. In such a case, all group members, including the resistive ones, must still agree on the dreamage. There are many life situations where no one likes a compromise but all believe the compromise is better than available alternatives. As a general rule, the W. C. Fields Principle of Dreamage Creation holds true: "*If at first you don't succeed, try, try again. Then give up. There's no use in being a damn fool about it.*" Although peace, love, and harmony are honorable ideals, they have a way of expressing themselves in their own time and place, often without regard to our waking preferences. Don't try to force it.

Generally speaking, a dreamage is constructive when the needs of all your interviewed characters are reflected by it. However, your Dream Self, which generally reflects your waking preferences, must agree to the dreamage and feel comfortable with it as well. After all, you must feel comfortable with a dreamage if you are to choose to work with it before sleep each night and during the day. Your own waking sense of inner and outer change in your life will help you to determine the usefulness of any particular dreamage as it is used.

Steps in dreamage construction

- Review the recommended dream changes in the Dream Commentary. If there is agreement, rewrite the original dream.
- Use as many of the original dream elements as possible. Include all interviewed characters unless one has stated it wants to be left out and all its fellows have no objection.
- Include all of the recommended dream changes in the dreamage.
- If an interviewed character does not support the changes desired by its fellows, respect its resistance. This is a fundamental form of deep listening and to do otherwise is to discount a perspective that clearly feels strongly enough about these things to be willing to hold out against its peers.

Criteria for dreamage construction

As indicated above, a well-constructed dreamage will usually contain *all* of the originally questioned interviewed characters but in a relationship which they themselves choose and agree upon as a group. This implies that all of the original perspectives, opinions, perspectives, and purposes embodied as interviewed characters will be retained, but reorganized to function in a more harmonious fashion. To do otherwise would be to repress or ignore aspects of self. In some cases, there will be a consensus that some interviewed character may not be included. As mentioned above, in such a case, *providing the interviewed character itself agrees*, it may be excluded from the dreamage.

Drawing from the suggestions of Kant, the dreamage may even contain rebellious and passionate activity as long as it is capable of being universalized to represent norms by which other interviewed characters can harmoniously live. For example, the *Bhagavad Gita* presents some warfare as in accordance with *dharma*. Discover morality within and externalize that moral example in the dreamage.

A potential ideal for every interviewed character is to be of service to its fellow interviewed characters. This perspective is summarized very well in a statement from the Cayce readings: *Know that the purpose for which each soul enters a material experience is that it may be a light unto others.*[8] However you frame your purpose or ideal, you will perceive and create reality in that context, so its formulation is not to be taken lightly. Each interviewed character (and dreamer) has the right to reject any ideal and the value system that it represents.

Unless the dream is its own dreamage, the dreamage will *not* contain all of the original actions and feelings occurring in most dreams. Altering perceived relationships inevitably alters actions and feelings, creating a new reality for the dreamer and fundamentally changing his or her perspective toward the life issues addressed by the dream or life drama. If you think of interviewed characters as conveyors of certain perspectives, actions and feelings, healing exists when these are in proper relationship.[9] In addition, when compared with the message of the original dream narrative, it is possible that the reality expressed metaphorically by the dreamage sends a different message to the cells of the body.

If all the interviewed characters in a dream or life drama are not interviewed, as is usually the case, the dreamage may not include important perspectives. In such cases, construct the dreamage, but with the recognition that it may represent a skewed portrayal of the needs of the group as a whole. If the interviewed characters have no objection, you may add interviewed characters to the Dream Commentary and to the dreamage that were not in the original dream narrative but that appear in the Dream Sociomatrix Commentary. In that case, summarize the Dream Commentary into a coherent narrative that structurally parallels the original dream narrative.

Here is the dreamage for *Ken Wilber Dies:*

> Ken Wilber and his girlfriend are killed in a head-on car crash. I am very upset. Ken, his girlfriend, their car, the other car, the other driver and myself are all terribly pissed. Some of us indulge in a bit of guilt and self-blame that we allowed this terrible thing to happen. But then we realize that we are all still alive enough to be pissed, so we must not be so dead after all! Now we are figuring out what we need to do to avoid these wrecks in the future. We decide to pray for other drivers and to feel that intent creating mental clarity and purity. We start to get in our cars to continue our lives, but then we decide, after we get to talking, that we are all going in the same basic direction instead of opposite directions. We decide to continue on together in some mutually chosen direction.

This dreamage would not work for you if you had the same dream. It may sound contrived or as just one more waking projection onto the dream, and indeed, for you it may very well be so. Whether you like it or not is not only irrelevant, it is counterproductive to attempt to make such evaluations. Your responsibility is to produce dreamages that *your* interviewed characters can support wholeheartedly. They will not be perfect, just as this one is not, but by using them you are subordinating your waking picture of integration and harmony to a broader, collective one. This will evoke and lead to clearer and yet more integrative and harmonious dreamages.

Over time you will develop a collection of dreamages that deal with finances, health, career decisions, interpersonal relationships, transpersonal development, and other areas of your life. You may want to keep your dreamage cards with you as you move through your day. When you find yourself in a life situation that is not to your liking, pull out an appropriate card. You may be angry, sad, scared, or confused. Find a card that is related to your current feelings as well as to the life issue at hand. Read over the dreamage, doing your best to experience it as if you are in the dreamage. By doing so, you are affirming integration and coherence on an experiential level in a way that speaks for your broader constituency much better than do mere thoughts or warm and fuzzy affirmations.

This general procedure is also recommended before sleep as an aid in the constructive programming of your dreams. In the five to 15 minutes in which you are drifting off to sleep you are at the most suggestible period of your 24-hour cycle. This slow dropping of waking awareness is called the hypnogogic state. It is the best time to restructure your awareness and program your dreams by experiencing a dreamage or two, ideally those related to life issues which you desire to incubate. Always put yourself *in* the dreamage. Experience it as real. Feel the emotions the images convey. Be your Dream Self. See and feel the other interviewed characters. Experience the events as happening *now*. Your willingness to do so will have a direct effect on the consciousness in which you enter sleep, positively affecting the context in which you dream, which will, in turn, affect how quickly themes of drama, in which you are persecuted or experience yourself as a victim, are neutralized. You may be surprised at the originality and creativity your interviewed characters subsequently display in metaphorically healing the life issues confronting you. This is a powerful movement away from drama and toward the lucidity embodied by broader collective and integrative contexts.

When you find that a dreamage has turned stale and no longer evokes the numinous presence of the dream, it often helps to read over the original Dream Sociomatrix Commentary to reawaken a sense of those perspectives involved in the life issue. Then too, new dreams will present reformulations of the same life issues but in terms relevant to the present.

A well-structured dreamage, when worked with properly, can be a powerful, healing force because images are personifications not only of preferences but of underlying intention and world views. Thoughts are things. They create our reality. Edgar Cayce made this point clearly to one person who, in a reading, asked him if her physical difficulties had any relationship to an accident that occurred many years previously. The response was that it affected her "*only so much as the mind allows self to associate same with the accident. For, as we have indicated, the body renews itself according to the mental perspective it holds toward ideals and in the light of the application of relationships to others. And this applies as well in the relationships to self.*" (Cayce, 2081–2) The dreamage is a form of "application of relationships" regarding internal "others."

Steps in dreamage application

1   Write out the dreamage agreed upon by your interviewed group members. Give it an original, catchy name, related to the name of the original dream, to help you both remember it and its relationship to the original dream, followed by a "D" to indicate "Dreamage."
2   Before sleep, read over the changed dream. Visualize the dreamage unfolding exactly as if you are asleep, dreaming it. Put as much feeling into the experience as possible. Do this several times.
3   When you anticipate life situations that involve the life issue addressed by the intrasocial group, such as an argument or feelings of loneliness or abandonment, pull out your note card and imagine yourself in the situation of the dreamage as you read the card. Observe what subsequently occurs in the situation.
4   If you have dreams or waking events that you think reflect the influence of your dreamage, indicate the connection on a note card, dating your entry, and filing it with the dreamage note card. This will help you to assess the impact of the dreamage on your life.

Dreamages and dream manipulation

Is the construction of a dreamage simply a way of extending waking autocratic control over new inner dominions? This is a concern that has led some dream researchers to the conclusion that a dream should not be changed. While it is indeed possible to alter the dream process to bend it to waking will in various ways, as is common with lucid dreaming, to do so does not reflect the purposes of IDL. Robert H. Jackson, the chief US prosecutor at the Nuremburg trials, agrees: "Those who begin coercive elimination of dissent soon find themselves exterminating dissenters. Compulsory unification of opinion achieves only an unanimity of the graveyard."[10] Respect for the autonomy of interviewed emerging potentials requires that you consult your interviewed characters prior to changing those intentions and preferences that the interviewed characters personify. While doing so is certainly not required – you do so without thought whenever you take waking action – opening a dialogue with these invested perspectives implies that you are willing to listen to their needs. To do otherwise is to discount perspectives, a choice for which you may pay by increased internal conflict or reduced future contact. As Mary Cassatt has wisely observed, acceptance on someone else's terms is worse than rejection. If you expect other perspectives to accept you as you are, equity requires that you strive to accept them as they are.

There is nothing inherently dysfunctional about changing dreams – as long as you are not simply imposing a tighter degree of waking authoritarianism upon your intrasocial reality. If you do not wish to inadvertently generate more conflict it would be wise to accept and respect emerging potentials by taking them into account in your interventions. Again, keeping an eye open for dream feedback is helpful in this regard.

A common criticism of dreamages that is heard is, "Can't one resistant group member block the will of the majority?" "Isn't this encouraging a form of internal totalitarianism?" There are several responses to this criticism. If you go ahead and ignore the resistance of perspectives, you are repressing conflict. This is counter to the intent of IDL. Conflict at subliminal levels is occurring continuously at *thesis* levels of development; conscious conflict is a necessary attribute of the *antithesis* stage, necessary for higher-order integration and transformation as *synthesis*.

Part of the normal function of waking consciousness is to make unilateral decisions without taking into account intrasocial consensus. This is the role of Dream Self fulfilling its function as confident leader regarding relationships with the world. In many decisions, there naturally exists some ambivalence, which means there are generally invested perspectives that disagree with your course of action. We can tell their presence by feelings of doubt or confusion or by resistance to change or by a desire for chocolate instead of vegetables or fruit. If we waited until we had complete consensus in life, there are few things that we would ever accomplish. Consequently, IDL encourages you to trust and support waking identity its decision making most of the time, but occasionally consult its broader constituency to verify that its direction is moving toward closer alignment with the priorities of one's life compass.

IDL is a "time out" from business as usual. It is like getting a checkup at the doctor's office and getting your blood taken so you can assess the balance of various metabolic processes. It is a time when you set aside your normal waking agenda in order to consult the priorities of your broader intrasocial community. It can prevent the imposition of a dreamage on the group if one is not warranted. This is not bad modeling for waking life, since history is filled with instances of the imposition of the will of one individual or group on others. If consensus building as a pre-requisite to dreamage creation teaches us to listen to resistance, we have learned an important skill that may help reduce the tendency to impose our will and ignore the resistance of others in our waking lives.

Summary

• Creating dreamages is practice at establishing internal governance based on consensus.
• Consensus internal governance is much more likely to reflect your overall needs regarding healing, balance, and transformation than is the autocratic rule of only one aspect of yourself, your waking identity.

- Using dreamages is a way to tell yourself that you are attempting to set your own agenda aside in favor of a more broad-based, intrinsic approach to resolving your life issues.

Notes

1 Shepherd, C. R. (1964). *Small Groups: Some Sociological Perspectives.* San Francisco: Chandler, p. 25.
2 Bales, R. F. (1950). *Interaction Process Analysis.* Cambridge, MA: Addison-Wesley, p. 61.
3 This is probably an infinite regress. You will never reach a *maximum* positive impact because no matter how many emerging potentials you incorporate into your expanding sense of self, no matter how many perspectives you consult, there will always remain relatively disenfranchised ones.
4 I am not suggesting that the dreamage is created as spontaneously as is a dream. It is not, but it is arguably closer in origin to innate processes than a waking construct which is a product of waking identity rather than a collective and intrasocial creation.
5 Bateson, G. (1975). *Steps to an Ecology of Mind.* New York: Ballantine. Bateson's concept of schismogenesis involves a growing split in the structure of human interaction and in the ideas communicated about it.
6 Dream group distributions as depicted in the Dream Sociogram fall into three basic categories, thesis, antithesis, and synthesis. Thesis patterns reflect attempts to maintain the *status quo* and functional balance in the face of conflict. Antithesis patterns reflect deeper conflict that undercuts basic self-acceptance. Synthesis patterns reflect interviewed character mutual agreement and acceptance. There are two sub-categories. These are high synthesis, in which interviewed character preferences are consistently very positive, and nightmare antithesis patterns, in which destructive choosing perspectives prevail in consciousness, forcing normally accepting emerging potentials to be rejecting. All of these are explained in depth in *Understanding the Dream Sociogram.*
7 A disenfranchised perspective is oppressed, most likely by waking totalitarianism; an impulsive perspective is likely an addiction in the role of persecutor in the Drama Triangle.
8 Cayce, E. (1972). *Readings.* Virginia Beach, VA: ARE Press, pp. 641–646.
9 Master K'ung (Confucius) would say that they reflect *the will of heaven.*
10 Excerpts of Court's Ruling On Compulsory Oath to Flag. *New York Times,* August 27, 1988.

Bibliography

Bales, R. F. (1950). *Interaction process analysis.* Cambridge, MA: Addison-Wesley.
Bateson, G. (1975). *Steps to an ecology of mind.* New York: Ballantine.
Cayce, Edgar. (1972). *Readings.* Virginia Beach, VA: A.R.E. Press.
Shepherd, C. R. (1964). *Small groups: Some sociological perspectives.* San Francisco: Chandler.

Chapter 21

Creating the Waking Commentary

> We should honor our teachers more than our parents, because while our parents cause us to
> live, our teachers cause us to live well.
>
> Philoxenus

As teachers and molders of personality, your dream characters can have as profound effect upon you as do your parents, whether or not you remember your dreams. The Waking Commentary will teach you to use the recommendations of your interviewed characters to make concrete, powerful improvements to your life.

Purpose of the Waking Commentary

During the storms of life, a submarine can be very useful. As Joseph Chilton Pearce said,

> Problem-solving is like patching holes in a rotten boat; for each patch applied, two
> more leaks spring up. There are times when a way out is needed that is not available
> to logical patching techniques. There are times when we need a way beyond rotten
> hulks, a way not for restructuring a new boat or even a serviceable life-jacket, but
> rather some sub-mariner's way through a sea of confusion to new terrain.

Interviewed characters from your dreams and life dramas are like submarines, taking novel and creative viewpoints toward those issues in your life where you are stuck or asleep. If you have the courage to implement their suggestions in your waking life, you will be impressed with how previously impassible roadblocks fade away or at least become manageable.

In the Waking Commentary, each interviewed character listed in the Dream Sociomatrix asks itself the following questions,

> If I were this dreamer and lived her waking life for her, how would I live it differently?
> Would I handle her three life issues differently? If so, how?

Answers are written in the Waking Commentary for several purposes. It is important to indicate to your intrasocial community that you respect it and are interested in doing more than gaining insight into your dreams or life dramas. Inner cooperation and support is more forthcoming if you demonstrate a commitment to use the information gleaned from your dialogues with emerging potentials. The relevance of intrasocial groups to waking concerns is strengthened through your attention and application. Waking Commentary elaborations are evidential in that they demonstrate the relevancy of the Dream Sociometric process to your ongoing life concerns.

Each interviewed character's responses are noted. You can then decide the merit of what is said and choose to either ignore or act on the suggestions made. You decide which, if any, of the recommendations you would like to implement in your daily life. Those suggestions that represent the strongest group consensus are probably the most important and will receive the most support throughout the change process.

Interviewed character responses to the second question ("Would you handle my three life issues differently?") provide an opportunity for intrasocial sources of objectivity to provide their perspectives regarding issues of concern to you in your daily life. Most people report these recommendations are practical and useful, taking dreamwork and self-development out of the realm of insight and into the domain of pragmatic relevancy.

Alternative ways to ask the Waking Commentary questions

Some people have a difficult time understanding these questions when they first encounter them. Some respond with a dream change, while others imagine that they are the interviewed character, say, a crocodile, trying to live their waking life rather than being the perspective embodied as the crocodile. Alternative wordings may be helpful:

- *If I were _____ (the dreamer) in her waking life and had to make her decisions about career, work, finances, relationships, transpersonal development, health, would I do anything differently? If so, what?*
- *If I were the life compass of this dreamer and made all of his waking decisions for him, would any of my choices be different? If so, which ones? Why?*
- *If _____ (the dreamer) thought, felt and acted the way I do, how would her life be different?*

Thinking of the interviewed character as a muse who is being given the opportunity to run the drama of everyday life is helpful for some people.

While most people do an excellent job of answering this question once they grasp it, there are sometimes abstract concerns that bear mentioning. Some people are afraid that fragmentation, decompensation, or dissociation is encouraged by this question. But such processes are involuntary while the stepping aside of waking identity that is encouraged in IDL is voluntary. This simple distinction makes all the difference. Practice in *choosing* to observe your life from another internally legitimate perspective builds your sense of who you are while expanding it.

The Waking Commentary question and elaborations

There are five steps in the procedure of creating the Waking Commentary:

1) First become the interviewed character that follows Dream Self in the left-hand margin list of choosers in the Dream Sociomatrix. Ask, as (this interviewed character): *if I were living this dreamer's waking life, how would I live it differently? Would I handle this dreamer's three life issues differently? If so, how?*
2) Write responses following the Dream Commentary.
3) Repeat this procedure with each subsequent interviewed character and *Dream Consciousness*, then ending with Dream Self.
4) Write a summary statement of the life changes that the interviewed characters encourage you to make, being as specific as possible.
5) Decide which recommendations you think are beneficial and reasonable.

Example: The Waking Commentary for *Ken Wilber Dies* is as follows:

Ken Wilber:	Knowing what I know now, I would tell the dreamer not to worry about killing me. He can't. I would also tell him to continue to practice listening deeply to himself. That cultivates the witness within him in a moment-to-moment way in his daily life more than meditation does and I know what I'm talking about, because I'm a champion meditator! (But don't get me wrong – I'm not suggesting that he not meditate! On the other hand, you will benefit greatly from practicing at every opportunity!) The weight you want to lose will take care of itself as you learn to listen to your body and to respect what it says it wants and doesn't want.
Girlfriend:	Nothing to add!
Car:	Sounds good to me!
Second Car:	Stop blaming yourself for screwing up!
Other Driver:	Agreed!
Dream consciousness:	Sounds like good advice. I would review the dreamage.
Dream Self:	OK!

Notice that this Ken Wilber is saying things that the *real* Ken Wilber would not say. Because Wilber is unfamiliar with IDL, he would not advocate deep listening over meditation. Even if he was familiar with IDL, he would be unlikely to place a discipline that is anchored in the subtle as higher than a discipline that at best is anchored in the causal and non-dual.[1]

Recommendations are sometimes provided as dream metaphors. For example, slowing down the hectic pace of one's life may be expressed as "taking your foot off the accelerator," or "downshifting." Such metaphorical allusions are not unusual in Dream Sociometry, and you will often find such statements in the comments of characters if you interview others or read their interviews. When you keep track of what these interviewed characters personify, you are teaching yourself to think metaphorically about life.

Summary

- The Waking Commentary provides specific recommendations for changing your life. These may be perspectival, attitudinal, emotional, or behavioral.
- These recommendations demonstrate the relevance of IDL to issues that are central to your life or that of your students.

Note

1 It is not unusual in IDL to encounter dream characters and the personifications of life issues that present and amplify causal perspectives. These are seen in identification with the perspective of Dream Consciousness, in the occasional appearance of transpersonally neutral preferences and through identification with perspectives that are clearly formless and possess no sense of self whatsoever. However, because IDL involves a sophisticated use of imagery for the purpose of transcendence of imagery, it is still imagery based, which makes it at best a high subtle level yoga. Meditation, however, is at its best clearly anchored in the formless, and meditators will find a greater number of formless perspectives in their IDL interviews.

Chapter 22

The Identification Commentary

The purpose of the Identification Commentary is to pinpoint specific life circumstances in which to practice a core application of IDL: identification with an interviewed character for a transformational purpose. When combined with a core practice of IDL, deep listening, identification hastens the expression of the qualities of your life compass in your daily life.

The theory is simple. If there are perspectives that have clearly demonstrated, both through their preferences and their elaborations, that they are more accepting, more compassionate, more wise, and more at peace than you are, then identification with them in those situations where they think they can make the most difference in your life puts them, IDL, and your desire for personal transformation to the test.

The Identification Commentary

The purpose of the Identification Commentary is to determine specific waking life circumstances in which an interviewed character recommends that you become it and live your life as if *they* were running the show. The question is,

> *(Interviewed character,) in what life situations would it be most beneficial for me to imagine that I am you and act as you would?*

Another way of asking this question is:

> *If I could designate specific occasions in the dreamer's waking life when I would recommend that he imagine that he is me, what would those occasions be?*

The more specific and clear the circumstances are in which you are to identify with this or that interviewed character, the better.

Here are some examples of some interviewed character recommendations for waking identification:

Grand Piano: Become me whenever you need to feel in balance and in harmony. I am those things, so when you are me,

	you will project those qualities. When you play piano would be a good time to identify with me! So would teaching.
Observatory:	Become me when you need perspective, detachment and ability to witness. When you are meditating, for instance.
Wolf:	Whenever you want to feel alive! Particularly during the chest part of inhalation during meditation.
Man:	(Riding a bucking piano and playing it.) Whenever you feel out of balance, strung out, you can be me and you will be identified with a perspective that can ride the bronco of your life. For example, when you are feeling challenged and are needing to take risks.
Dream Consciousness:	Be me when you want to cultivate an ability to witness all thoughts, all images, all form, particularly when you meditate.
Richard Gere:	I most closely personify the part of you that is transpersonally adept, yet successful in the world. I have fame and fortune in addition to a transpersonal discipline of some significance. The reason why I am in this dream is to help you to claim me as a significant and genuine part of yourself. If you will imagine that you are me, you will internalize those attributes that I possess that you lack.

As you can see, there are overlapping recommendations. A number of these interviewed characters are interested in enhancing this dreamer's mediations. They reflect different perspectives, each of which brings helpful awakenings to practice. The dreamer can use different ones at different times during his meditations.

The recommendations for identification from *Ken Wilber Dies* are:

| *Ken Wilber:* | Become me when you want to cultivate your ability to witness, particularly to gain some objectivity from your addictions in order to become aware of them dispassionately as an aid to their transformation. |

As you develop a repertoire of identifications, develop a chart. These interviewed characters become members of your ongoing IDL intrasocial Sangha. Write the interviewed character's name and beside it the circumstances in which it recommends that you become it. Students have reported "magical" healing of relationships, life circumstances, and health conditions using this procedure. Put it to the test in your life! While the following examples do not begin to convey the power of this process, you can at least get a sense of how you can chart these special interviewed characters and the life circumstances in which you desire their assistance.

Chart 22.1

Interviewed character	Situation/Life Issue for Identification
Plywood	When having conversations with Clark; anytime feeling guilty about things that I may have done wrong
School Bus	When I feel there is a lot of confusion that I can't get out of
Baby	When I am having trouble trusting, when there is a twinge of self-doubt
Red Rocks	In the morning when I usually feel frazzled and unstructured. I can use them to feel structured.
Razor Blade	Become me when you want a clearer reality of your workplace. You will know that your intent is good, have confidence that what you have is what it takes, and walk through each day without anxiety.
Sea	When I am in charge of your life, you have no anxiety. I know how to go with the flow. I am not afraid of death. There is no death. It's vast.

Summary

- Identifying with interviewed characters that personify attributes of your life compass increases the likelihood that you will respond in a healthy manner in important life situations.
- Develop a chart to keep track of who to identify with in what life situation.

Chapter 23

Designing your Action Plan

The Action Plan

(All of these recommendations for waking life applications are not necessarily helpful or of equal importance. You have to decide how you wish to prioritize them and what you want to do with them. But take some action! It is a way of demonstrating that you take your inner direction seriously. If you have it wrong, future dream groups will cybernetically correct your course.)

Listening deeply to dream and life drama perspectives evolves awareness. As C. G. Jung has said,

> *In each one of us there is another whom we do not know. He speaks to us in dreams and tells us how differently he sees us from how we see ourselves. When we find ourselves in an insolubly difficult situation, this stranger in us can sometimes show us a light which is more suited than anything else to change our perspective fundamentally, namely just that perspective which had led us into the difficult situation.*[1]

Each interview is an incubator of consciousness, a bridge between waking awareness and formless wellsprings of creativity. As such, interviewing functions in a way similar to myths of cosmology or creation, providing metaphorical models for your habits and your actions. While identification with interviewed emerging potentials in specific life situations is perhaps the most important action you can take in IDL, you will find within the various commentaries many other recommendations for the resolution of your life issues. What are you to do with these?

You can relieve the suffering intrinsically associated with identification with habit in any number of ways. You can focus on *action*, using behavior modification or lifestyle alterations: exercise, diet, communication skills; you can do types of body work to break up and change somatic and affective patterns; you can focus on *affect* by using such methods as Gestalt therapy or play therapy; you can intervene in your *thought processes* with cognitive therapy, Rational Emotive Therapy, Reality Therapy, or Transactional Analysis; you can emphasize *life purpose and transpersonal growth* by focusing on meditation, values, psychosynthesis, or your particular religious mythology; you can even intervene out of awareness through suggestion, hypnotherapy, biofeedback, prayer, neurotechnology, and dreamwork. Each of us is more responsive to some of these approaches and less responsive to others. Therapists tend to use and to be most effective with those approaches that personally fit for them. A balanced integral life practice will generate a program that addresses all of these different areas.

The *Action Plan* for your Dream Sociogram involves the determination of what, if any, interviewed character recommendations you deem worth implementing in your daily life. It summarizes interviewed character recommendations made in all the commentaries.

All of the above recommendations for waking life application are not of equal importance. You have to decide how you wish to prioritize them and what you want to do with them. But take some action! Doing so is a way of demonstrating that you respect and trust at least some of your interviewed emerging potentials. If you have it wrong, future dream and life drama sociomatrices will cybernetically correct your course.

List all the recommendations you find in all the commentaries. Decide which ones are important to you. Prioritize them by placing numbers before them. Create a daily self-monitoring structure that will allow you to observe what changes you are making and understand what resistances you are encountering. Here were the recommendations from *Ken Wilber Dies:*

> regular review of life application of my Action Plan
> review of this reading
> regular meditation
> pre-sleep incubation of my dreamage (if any)
> pre-sleep incubation of some particular life issue, asking for support of appropriate dream group members.

remembering to identify with confident, capable dream group members at specific waking moments, such as when needing more self-acceptance or courage or patience, etc. (Write a list of specific situations where identification with one or another particular dream group member will be particularly helpful, then review how you did at the end of the day.)

Not to worry about killing myself because I can't!

Continue to practice listening deeply to myself to cultivate the moment-to-moment witness in my daily life.

Continue practicing meditation, perhaps with the frame of mind of this Dream Consciousness in mind.

Listen to my body regarding food preferences.

Continue to practice being thankful for other drivers.

I want to take on reviewing the dreamage and practicing being Dream Consciousness at different times during the day, particularly when I am meditating or worried about my weight.

Some of the basic issues addressed by this dream group are

- Don't take myself so seriously!
- When I screw up, don't waste time beating myself up. It's grandiose to feel so responsible or irresponsible!
- Practice thankfulness and appreciation in small ways.

Subsequent Dream Sociomatrices and interviews will help you to evaluate the effectiveness of your Action Plan. If you receive strong but extreme recommendations from one interviewed character, it is wise to get feedback from other interviewed characters that you respect. This happens automatically with Dream Sociometry. Such feedback does not have to come from the same dream or waking drama. Growth is a cybernetic or self-correcting process. As you act on character suggestions, you will receive subsequent feedback from other interviewed characters.

Perhaps the most important way to evaluate your application is the usefulness of interviewed character suggestions in moving toward resolution of your life issues. Sometimes it is sufficient to understand the process from the perspective of your life compass. That way, you are less likely to feel that you are a victim of circumstances. At other times, you will experience issues that had long plagued you melting away, either in importance or in actuality.

It is also recommended that you share your course of action with people who you trust who can provide additional help. However, exercise caution. It is not unusual to want to share exciting new insights indiscriminately. That can create unnecessary problems if the ground has not been prepared. People may not understand or in one way or another undercut your Action Plan. Consider your own need for the approval or acceptance by others. Sharing dream information can put you in a vulnerable position with some insecure or ignorant people. Remember that your blood family is not the same as your transpersonal family, although the two may overlap. Do not try to gain validation and support from people who do not have the background or interest to provide either.

Steps in the development of your Action Plan

- Write out, as specifically as possible, the changes you wish to make in your life based not only on the Waking Life Commentary but on life change recommendations that you may have received in the other commentaries.

An interviewed character from a dream, a hatchet, recommended that it be turned into a vajra, a Tibetan symbol of diamond-knowledge and thunderbolt-like enlightenment. It suggested that the dreamer hold one during meditation. "I cut through things, but aggressively. As a *vajra*, I cut through things like diamond, like a lightening bolt. I am the mind you want in your journey." "Discernment and clarity in writing and meditation are my gifts. Keep me with you!"

The Action Plan was to meditate holding the vajra, as an affirmation that its qualities were being amplified in consciousness.

Troubleshooting your Action Plan

> *You can judge your age by the amount of pain you feel when you come in contact with a new idea.*
>
> John Nuveen

There are several possible reasons why you may not follow through with your Action Plan.

Set goals that motivate you

Different priorities continually compete for your attention. You will have to choose repeatedly between new, desirable, but relatively unrooted behaviors that you are monitoring and older, less desirable, but much more powerfully ingrained habits. Your goals need to be important enough to you to stick with them. It's just as difficult to reach a destination you've never seen as it is to come back from a place you've never been. Choose goals that not only your interviewed characters think are important, but that *you* are motivated to attain. Choose behaviors that you *want* to change, not that you *need* to change or that you *should* change. To strengthen your new behaviors, keep your goals and your purpose in your thoughts. Repeating to yourself what you want to accomplish and why before you go to bed and first thing in the morning can make a huge difference in terms of your focus on your chosen priorities. Reviewing the Waking Life Commentary will help to increase your understanding of your purpose. It will also help keep the Action Plan high in your subliminal list of priorities.

What's your payoff?

Measurable benefits that are necessary to provide you with motivation for continuing your waking application may not be great enough. What can you do to increase the amount of satisfaction that you derive from implementing your Action Plan? One dependable reward is the acknowledgement of a IDL peer, Practitioner, or Elder. Be sure to make use of them.

What are you up against?

When we attempt to establish new behaviors, we seldom consider that we have very good, very entrenched reasons for maintaining our old, comfortable behaviors. The general psychological term for these benefits, largely unrecognized, are "secondary gains." This refers to benefits we receive from not changing, staying stuck, sick or dysfunctional. If these reasons are not recognized, understood, and counteracted, you can do all the interviews in the world with the most wonderful emerging potentials and odds are that you will stay stuck. Therefore, it is important that you ask yourself the following questions: "Why haven't I changed this behavior before?" "Based on my past experience, how am I likely to sabotage the change I want to make?" "What is my plan for dealing with these self-defeating behaviors?" If you do not address these questions it probably is a sign that you aren't ready to take on a particular goal, that your desire to do so is an expression of hope, not commitment. In that case, it is wiser to drop that goal and pick another. You just aren't ready.

Set measurable goals

How are you going to know if you are making progress if you do not have some way of measuring your growth? How do you know when you're caring? What does it mean to be patient? When? How? What thoughts or feelings are associated with guilt? What does it mean to give yourself credit? Is this about any kind of sex, or just certain types? What does demonstrating physical affection mean concretely? If you are looking for improvements in your relationship with your father, how are you going to measure the change? Fewer arguments? More smiles? More positive, supportive statements?

Decide what changes you are going to measure. Many of the changes in IDL are seen in particular circumstances, for example, in an improvement in your relationship with a family member. What is going to be different tomorrow than it was today? How are you going to know? Choose observable changes for which improvement can be measured in a short period of time – one hour, one day, one week. If you can't measure a change you are basing your life on hope and wishful thinking.

Be realistic!

Your Action Plan may be too complicated or ambitious. If so, re-evaluate it. Do you need to set smaller, more specific and attainable sub-goals? Improve your Action Plan until you can reach some daily goal comfortably.

You may find that you have quite a few recommendations to sort through, prioritize, and choose among. Do not overload yourself by attempting to make too many changes at one time. Be realistic in what you expect yourself to do, limiting yourself to one or two lifestyle changes at a time, emphasizing those that seem to be most persistently recommended and that you agree with. For example, if you find repeated recommendations for you to meditate regularly, then you might want to move that to the top of your IDL "to do" list in your Action Plan. Acting on the recommendation toward which you feel the most resistance will free the most energy for the completion of other items on your list.

Allow time for change

How much time will be required to accomplish the life changes you want? Most change programs require a minimum of a month to six weeks before the new behavior takes hold as a habit. Even then, there remains the possibility that an extinguished behavior, like smoking, will reassert itself in a moment when vigilance is down. Many people are enticed by six-day diets and seven-day stop-smoking programs. The truth of the matter is that you need to ask yourself a very basic and important question before you attempt to implement any intrasocial group based application plan: *am I ready and willing to commit myself to this new behavior for the rest of my life? Am I willing to give this new behavior priority over other changes I desire until it has become a natural part of my life?* In a very real sense, then, it is wise to expect any behavior change you wish to undertake will be a lifetime effort requiring some level of sustained vigilance.

In order to overcome unexpected resistances and obstacles, re-evaluate your Action Plan on a weekly basis. Commit yourself to as much time as you need to form new habit patterns: a month, three months, or six months. Be flexible with yourself by reappraising the appropriateness of your efforts on a weekly basis.

Get support!

Many people have difficulty asking for the help they need to make changes. If you aren't able to change, this is the first place to check – do you have enough support? You will need reinforcement and support to make lasting changes. What is your plan to obtain the support you will need? What type of support do you need? How often will you need support? For how long will you need to receive it? Will others welcome the change in your life or create static? Who can you talk to? What do you need to ask others to do for you?

You may tell yourself that you don't need support or that you *shouldn't;* you don't want to appear weak or think of yourself as dependent on others. You may feel that you are imposing and taking up the precious time of others for frivolous reasons that you should manage yourself. If so, consider how you feel when others ask you for support. Do you feel imposed upon? Generally, people feel honored and respected when they are asked for help and will do what they can to either help or point one toward sources that they have found helpful. Why wouldn't others do the same for you?

If you are not already a member of an ongoing IDL Sangha, seek one out or start an Integral Salon of your own. Check out "Friends of IDL" on Facebook for other students and Practitioners around the world for you to network with. Of course, the most important support that you can receive is the support that you give yourself. Your interviewed emerging potentials can be strong and constant allies in this regard.

Life change is challenging for us even when we are highly motivated. Put the odds in your favor by getting not only the ongoing support of your internal Sangha, but by embarking on a long-term student relationship with a Practitioner of IDL. Such a relationship provides ongoing accountability and objectivity from someone who understands your approach and is themselves practicing this work in their lives. The IDL coaching program is one way to do this: http://integraldeeplistening.com/become-an-idl-coach/

Prefer changes supported by a majority of your intrasocial community

Choose behavioral goals that seem to have the consistent support of a majority of characters that you have interviewed in different Dream Sociomatrices or individual interviews. This increases your internal support and decreases internal resistance.

When energy is directed into fundamental goals, secondary goals become easier to accomplish. Therefore, choose behavioral goals that seem to be fundamental. For instance, improving your health is a more fundamental goal than finding the right mate. Discovering and maintaining your peace of mind is a more fundamental goal than improving your health.

Be sure to check your priorities against those of your interviewed characters. Just because you think that a goal is fundamental, that does not mean that it is a priority of your intrasocial community. In the area of application, it is best to err on the side of cooperation with a broad intrasocial consensus.

When major interests are in opposition, such as seen in the dream *Equine Cannibals*, or where the pattern itself remains vague, such as in *Vicious Horses*, constructive change is more difficult. For change to occur, you don't have to *always* support the change. You only have to agree to the change at those crucial moments when choice is realistic. For instance, if you want to meditate regularly, it is not necessary that you want to meditate all the time, but only at that time in the day when it is actually time to meditate. Even at those moments, it is not necessary that every aspect of yourself want to meditate. Only 51% of your invested forces must agree to meditate, and *only* at those times when the decision to meditate is required. If your goal is to go out and take a jog, only 51% of your intention needs to be activated for you to put on your running shoes and go outside. You don't require 95% or 100% agreement, but only a simple majority. The more support that you receive for any course of action at those crucial moments, the easier any new behavior will be to maintain. Those moments are the times when you need to have internal Sangha members you can identify with and waking Sangha members you can lean on.

Don't forget to use dreamages and pre-sleep suggestions

Pre-sleep visualization of a dreamage is often a recommended part of the Action Plan. However, it will be rare that you will notice dramatic feelings when you review a dreamage before you go to sleep at night or at other times. Many medicines are subtle in their effect or require accumulated dosages to have an effect. Most are intended to alter awareness on the level of cell and organ physiology and only indirectly have an effect on waking awareness. Of course, the more that you emotionally and behaviorally identify with the action patterns in the dreamage, the more powerful the effect of the experience will be for you.

As you use pre-sleep suggestion, think of yourself as a sort of farmer of the mind who is planting seeds. If it is good seed, then it will bear fruit in season, provided the ground is suitable and there are proper proportions of sun and water. Be prepared to plant many seeds to overcome the inevitable weeds. The growth sequence is easier to plan for when it is understood. In a burnt-out forest clearing, weeds are the first life to return. In other words, without a clear set of life priorities, habitual thoughts and feelings will naturally take over your consciousness. If you set a clear agenda for yourself and "water" it, in time the psychological equivalent of bushes and scrub trees appear, followed by the longer growing, more sturdy hardwoods. As the hardwoods become taller their leaves create a canopy, filtering the light to the forest floor. If they are dense enough, weeds and most undergrowth are killed off, and the forest is returned to its natural equilibrium. If you plant "hardwood," you will eventually kill off your "weeds" naturally. Just as seeds germinate out of awareness below the ground, so dreamages do their work out of the light of the waking mind. It is enough for you, as a farmer of enlightenment, to have faith in the process, to plant your seeds and release them. Remember that the wise farmer or nurseryman does not plant more seed than he can cultivate, tend, and harvest. Focus on quality, not quantity. Focus on one or two dreamages rather than planting an endless variety.

Ask for and expect ongoing feedback from your dreams

Expect feedback in the form of subsequent dreams that comment on the new pattern of perspective and action that you are expressing. For instance, the dream *Learning to Fly* reflects the approval of interviewed characters for the effort at meditation by waking self – an activity recommended by earlier Action Plans. Expect an increase in both the quantity and quality of your dreams as you begin to put them to work in your life. Such cooperation will release powerful flows of intention as you integrate interests that were previously locked in conflict.

Listen to and respect resistance

Most resistance boils down to one fundamental perspective that we all share: we are not used to sharing power with intrasocial perspectives, and we don't like it. Perhaps we are afraid of "ego fragmentation," but more likely, we are comfortable running the show, just like most leaders. When it comes time to step down, most will work hard to maintain their power.

Assume that whatever recommendations are made by interviewed characters are the single most important changes which you can make to improve your life. This may not be true, but it is a good working proposition. Expect to encounter resistance, both from within yourself and from others as you change. You may think that the suggested changes are irrelevant, impractical, or foolish. This is partially because you already have your own list of priorities, your own agenda for self-improvement. It takes courage to change them simply upon the advice of some crazy interviewed characters.

Interior resistance will come from those perspectives that live off the secondary gains associated with your old habits and are made uncomfortable by your movement away from the *status quo*. Resistance will come from others who either have a comfortable image of who you are that they do not want to question or else are inconvenienced or made uncomfortable by your changes. For example, if they are used to drinking with you and you stop, that may make them more aware of their own drinking and their own motivations for continuing. It will be more comfortable for them if you just continue to drink.

Avoidance of recommendations due to discomfort, rationalization, apathy, guilt, fear of failure, or doubt is not unusual; accept such factors as part of your growth process even if you don't like them. Go easy on yourself; be persistent, and enjoy the growth challenge you have chosen for yourself.

Change creates resistance. Be prepared to meet up with dream characters that represent resisting constituencies. They will argue persuasively that you are being unfair or killing them! Listen to them. Love them. They have legitimate needs and concerns that need to be considered. In addition, you can always dialogue with the resistance itself. Resistance will appear in your dreams in forms that will help you to first understand and then defuse it.

Resistance can also spring from your own waking non-identification with the change, since you are not yet your emerging potentials. In addition, you currently identify with perspectives, at least in part, that prefer the *status quo*. In either case, the solution is to enhance the quality and quantity of your identification with those emerging potentials that support the change. When you work with a IDL Practitioner as a student, you identify with a personification of those interior perspectives that strongly support your awakening, lucidity and enlightenment.

You will have many dreams for which you will not create an Action Plan, and you will create Action Plans that you do nothing with. Learn to observe and accept your resistance without relapsing into drama of self-blame or hopelessness. Behavioral change is normally accompanied by desire to indulge in old behaviors. This desire diminishes as you repeat the new behavior. The more often that you practice it under a wide variety of circumstances, the sooner it will become a habit. Many habits require daily application for months or years to become permanent. But have faith; your interviewed characters will always be with you to support and direct you. Many of them want you to succeed as much, if not more, than you do.

Understand approach-avoidance conflict

A principle of psychology states that the farther you are from some desired goal the more desirable it seems; the closer you are to the desired goal the more resistance to change is likely to present itself. This is called approach-avoidance conflict. Let us you want to lose weight. When you first decide that it will be beneficial and make sense for you to take off some pounds your motivation is as high as it ever is likely to get. You are in "approach" mode. As you begin to actually change your behavior, that is, eat either less or stop eating foods you prefer in the amount and frequency you are used to, inner constituencies that were quiet before grow in strength. The closer that you come to attaining a desired goal the larger in importance that which you must give up becomes: your hunger, your sense of comfort, your fears of starvation. At some point, the constituencies of the *status quo* become so loud and the constituencies of change become so quiet that they are in practice "outnumbered." What was the majority has become the minority; what was the minority has become the majority. You switch into "avoidance" mode. Your internal constituencies that will lose power from the change get louder and louder, encouraging your relapse. When you understand and accept this natural source of resistance in implementing your Action Plan, you can accept it and be prepared to counteract it.

Evaluate your progress regularly

At the end of your period of application, assess your progress. Was your plan realistic? Did you stick to it? Did you receive any dream feedback about your Action Plan?

As mentioned above, most changes take at least a month to become habits. Monitor your application for a week. Evaluate your progress and make a decision whether to continue, alter, or discontinue the plan. Many of the interviewed character suggestions will be repeated, especially those that your current Action Plan does not address. You will find that some Action Plans are naturally superseded by subsequent intrasocial group recommendations. You will also find that if you do not act on a behavior strongly recommended by a intrasocial group that it will come up again and again in other Waking Commentaries and Action Plans.

Record your progress

Awareness promotes change. Keep a daily record to indicate your progress in implementing each new behavior. With the combination of internal support, a good Action Plan and a IDL Practitioner, you can make changes in your life that are fundamental and of lasting significance.

Summary

- Compile all of your interviewed character's recommendations.
- Emphasize quality over quantity by not attempting to make too many changes at one time.
- If a recommendation is thematic, that is, it is repeated again and again by a number of different interviewed characters in many different dreams, give it priority in your application.
- Expect resistance to change; recognize that many problem behaviors take repeated attempts at change before they dissolve.

Note

1 Jung, C. G. (1964). *Collected Works of C.G. Jung, Volume 10: Civilization in Transition.* Bollingen: Princeton University Press.

Chapter 24

The Dream Sociogram Commentary

While the Sociogram Commentary can be created at any point after the Dream Sociogram has been constructed, it is inserted at this point in the flow of the template. You may leave it out or complete it later if you prefer. The Dream Sociogram is discussed in the accompanying text, *Understanding the Dream Sociogram*. However, this section is included here because it deals with the interpretive comments that you, the dreamer, make as you evaluate the Dream Sociogram for a particular dream. These interpretive comments are thereby included in the Dream Sociomatrix template that is your record of your encounter with this particular intrasocial group.

The Dream Sociogram Commentary includes five topics. The first, "Overall Pattern," is your assessment of the interactional patterns created by the preferences of your interviewed characters. These patterns are related to one of four stages the developmental dialectic, thesis, antithesis, nightmare antithesis, and synthesis patterns. The particular pattern that you observe the Dream Sociogram is related to the particular life issues with which your intrasocial group is concerned. All of this is explained in the text, *Understanding the Dream Sociogram*.

The Sociogram Commentary

The Sociogram Commentary, which is comprised of interpretive comments that you make when you examine the Dream Sociogram, is divided into five parts. First, you comment on the Overall Pattern of the Sociogram. Then you comment on the patterns you observe on each of the four axes, the Acceptance, Form, Process, and Affect Axes.

The remaining four topics of Dream Sociogram evaluation concern the four number lines or "axes" upon which interviewed character preference totals are plotted. The "Acceptance Axis" addresses the relationships among your interviewed characters as preferring or rejecting perspectives. How accepting of yourself are you? Why? How rejecting of yourself are you? Why? This information can help you understand how to increase your self-acceptance and how to stop sabotaging your growth through self-rejection.

The "Form Axis" evaluates the relationships among your interviewed characters as preferred or rejected perspectives. You will find that some emerging potentials that are most accepting are themselves rejected. Why? Why is it that some of your most rejecting emerging potentials are sometimes the most preferred by the intrasocial group? How do such internal conflicts express themselves in your life in ways that complicate and sabotage your development? What do you need to do to reduce and eliminate such conflicts?

The "Process Axis" evaluates the relationships among the action elements in your intrasocial group. Your interviewed characters will, on the whole, prefer some actions over others. Why? What does the conflict among the most preferred actions and the most rejected actions say about behavioral conflicts in your life that you may or may not be aware of? What can you do to neutralize them so that they do not undermine your development?

The final section is the "Affect Axis." The emotional elements in your intrasocial group are more or less preferred by this intrasocial group. Why? If there is more than one emotional element, why is one more preferred than another? What does that say about the values of the intrasocial group? What does the opposition among the emotions in this intrasocial group say about inner conflict that may interfere with your growth?

Here is the Dream Sociogram Commentary for *Ken Wilber Dies* followed by the Dream Sociogram created by this group.

Overall Pattern: This is a strong antithesis pattern with a number of interviewed characters, both rejecting and rejected. It is not a nightmare antithetical pattern because the most nurturing members are still most accepting.

Acceptance Axis: Ken Wilber is the only accepting interviewed character. All others are rejecting. Dream Consciousness is most accepting, but it is not an interviewed character. The most rejecting interviewed character is *Second Car*, presumably because it feels highly victimized.

Form Axis: It is unusual to see a perspective rejected so strongly as is the one personified by "other driver." Multiple perspectives really don't like this thoughtless, sleepwalking, negligent, inattentive approach to life. Multiple perspectives also don't like the parts of my body that are breaking down and are culpable in my own self-destruction. It's obvious that Girlfriend and Ken Wilber are both Dream Self surrogates, reinforcing waking perspectives that create conflict. This teaches me to look beyond what values I associate with Ken Wilber, since he basically echoes my own, if I want to find integration within myself. That perspective doesn't hold the answer, which is an awareness I did not receive from my associations to or interpretations of the dream, although it rings true. This is an example of how we misinterpret and put our faith in individuals and ideals that are not representative of our inner compass. It suggests that we must eventually withdraw our unrealistic projections and expectations about them.

Process Axis: There is no bipolarity here, just widely condemned misbehavior and inattention. There is no internal conflict regarding behavior, because those actions identified in this group are all rejected!

Affect Axis: An uncomfortable behavior ("very upset") is preferred by this intrasocial group because it is appropriate to their circumstances, i.e., they identify strongly with victimization.

Summary

The purpose of the Dream Sociogram Commentary is to generate abstraction from scripting and drama through cultivating witnessing and objectivity

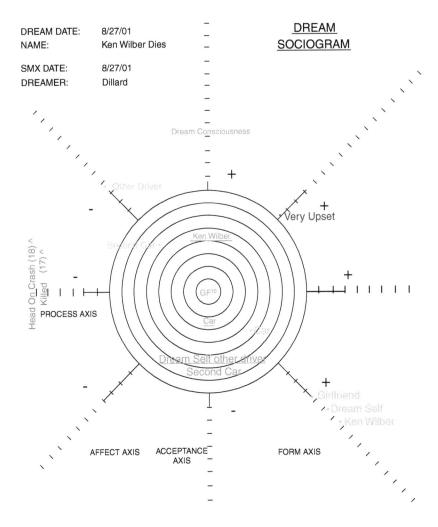

that transcends yet includes multiple relevant perspectives that together provide deeper and broader explanations for how you stay stuck and what you can do to stay unstuck.

The Dream Sociogram Commentary analyzes and interprets the patterns of intrasocial preference that are indicated in the Dream Sociomatrix.

It does so on four axes and in terms of various manifestations of the developmental dialectic.

Dream Sociogram interpretive comments help you to recognize how your patterns of intrasocial preference create conflict and harmony, fear and hope, confusion and wisdom within you.

Chapter 25

The Dream Group Dynamics Commentary

(In which the various interviewed characters are provided with an opportunity to express their thoughts on their relationships with their fellow interviewed characters.)

You have made your assessment of the Dream Sociogram. Your interpretive comments probably focus on the relationships among your various dream or life drama elements and their implications as seen from your perspective. But what of the interpretations of the Dream Sociogram by the other perspectives whose relationships are actually depicted in it? Following the Sociogram Commentary, your interviewed characters are given an opportunity to make their observations about your interpretations of the Sociogram in the Dream Group Dynamics Commentary. While some may have no opinions to offer, others will and those statements may be quite different from your own. Whose are more important, yours or theirs?

The purpose of this step is to provide both objectivity and feedback regarding your assessment of your intrasocial dynamics. You have drawn conclusions about what the Dream Sociogram is telling you, but it doesn't just represent you; it represents the interests of the other group members as well. What do they think of your interpretations? Since you will finally act on the basis of your own perspectives, you are well advised to take into account the perspectives of those characters that will be affected by your actions and whose support, or lack thereof, may determine the success of your efforts.

Here is the Dream Group Dynamics Commentary for *Ken Wilber Dies.*

Ken Wilber: We are not victims of anything but our own unrealistic expectations. If I blame the other driver, I blame that part of myself that he represents. That's foolish.

Girlfriend: I've got to learn to care big enough to stop caring the way I do! It's too personalized for my own good!

Car: Hey, cars come and they go. We're here to serve, but when it's time, just let us go!

Second Car:	We're imperfect. Don't lose too much sleep over it. Just factor it into your life and make the best of the ride.
Other Driver:	I am a part of you and therefore you are destined to screw up. So what? Let go of your unrealistic expectation that you will always be alert, aware, vigilant, discerning, etc. When you fall asleep, just learn from it, give thanks and go on.
Dream consciousness:	I really appreciate the time you took to learn from me.
Dream Self:	I give thanks to all these parts of myself for coming together and investing themselves for my greater good. Thank you!

Here is an example of comments made by members of another intrasocial group when asked to comment upon the Dream Sociogram that depicted their relationships:

Lois:	I am very glad to have Joe back and I have to say that I owe it to Joseph. So I appreciate it.
Room:	It really doesn't matter that I am plain and Lois thinks I am not. What matters is that she is happy. So don't try to fix her. Just make her feel supported.
House:	Agreed.
Door:	You are opening the doors to emerging potentials that want to be let in. Congratulations!
Dad:	I now have a much improved relationship with other aspects of my greater identity.
Couch:	What was missing is no more. I am where I am supposed to be and being used appropriately. Bringing Lois and Joe together allows you to get out of the hot seat. Metaphorically speaking, if you let the "Dad" part of yourself communicate with Mary Jane, your life will run a lot smoother.

Summary

- Unlike the other commentaries following the Dream Sociomatrix Commentary, you interpret the Dream Sociogram before your interviewed characters do. This is because waking identity is responsible for analyzing the Dream Sociogram and that information must be available before your interviewed characters can comment.

Chapter 26

What I am saying
to myself is . . .

Statements from elaborations are rewritten here as "I" statements

As you identified with this or that interviewed character, which expressed preferences and noted their elaborations in the various commentaries, some statements probably stood out as being particularly appropriate or important expressions of truth about who you are and your life circumstances. You were encouraged to underline them at that time rather than taking the time to ponder, interpret, or analyze them. This was to encourage you to stay in role as you worked through the experience of the dream or life drama from the perspective of this or that interviewed character.

Now is the time that you go back, find those underlined, statements and copy and paste them here. Now change them into "I" statements. You do this by changing the wording from a statement by an interviewed character to a comment you are telling yourself. After all, to the extent that your interviewed characters are parts of yourself, their statements are declarations that you are making about yourself and your life. "I" statements help you to take full responsibility for the implications of what you are telling yourself. Rewriting statements as "I" statements will also help you learn how to read back to students the statements made by characters during the single-character interviewing process.

Here are some examples of underlined character elaborations turned into "I" statements. The writing of "I" statements is followed by statements that summarize what you have learned from them.

Here are "I" statements for *Ken Wilber Dies*. They are adaptations of underlined statements found in the various commentaries.

"I am the instrument by which insensitivity and injustice occurs."

"I need to practice non-attachment, thankfulness, appreciation, moment to moment."

"I need to let go of the need to justify my existence."

"I need to drop my unrealistic expectations and my guilt when I don't live up to them."

"I need to let go of my fear of physical death so that I can live more courageously as I grow older."

"I need to learn compassion toward my own self-destruction."

"I need to gain objectivity toward the drama of my fears, my expectations, my self-blame."

"I need to let go of my sense of unfairness or injustice, particularly regarding my relationship with Mary Jane.

(In the following example, taken from commentaries accompanying another Dream Sociomatrix, these statements were made by a perspective which was bringing people back to life, but only partway, which was horrifying people.)

"I can bring them back partway. They have to bring themselves back the rest of the way. If you want to blame me because they aren't all the way back, OK, but you have to understand that people have to be willing to work to be reanimated. I can't and won't do it all for them."

"Dreaming only brings dead parts of myself part of the way back. They desire and need the continuing deep listening of IDL to bring them back completely. It is like rebirth. It will take commitment and effort for him to become fully living again."

"What I dislike most about being in this dream is that in order to get heard at all I have to first be perceived as the bad guy."

- I can bring myself back to life only partway. Dead parts of myself have to (be willing to) bring themselves back the rest of the way. If I want to blame myself because the dead parts of myself aren't all the way back, OK, but I have to understand that parts of myself have to be willing to work to be re-animated. I can't and won't do it all for them.
- It is like rebirth. It will take commitment and effort for me to become fully living again. Blaming myself because I am unaware of the fullness of these parts of myself is not helpful and it's not fair. Instead I need to focus on listening to them and identifying with them in order to fully bring them back to life.
- What I dislike most about my life is that in order to get heard at all I have to first be perceived as the bad guy. In order to be fully heard by myself and by others I feel I have to be willing to be perceived as the bad guy.
- I need to develop some compassion toward the part of myself which makes stupid choices unconsciously out of lack of discernment or unawareness because it is a natural part of myself and it will always be there.

What you do with such statements is of course up to you. However, to the degree that your "I! statements ring true for you, it is worth your time and energy to use them to act, think, or be different in your life today.

Summary

- "I" statements help you to take full responsibility for the implications of what you are telling yourself.
- Your elaborations of your "I" statements clarify and focus responsibilities that you are owning.

Chapter 27

The Dream Group Feedback Commentary

"Some of the basic issues addressed by this dream group are"

Your summary comments in this section will help you to get the big picture, to identify what you want to take with you out into the world and into tonight's sleep. It allows you to quickly grasp an overview of your work when you return to it, like an old friend, in years to come.

This section is also meant to help you to wake up, to keep from falling back asleep as much as you were before. It is not only easy but appallingly normal to forget, ignore, repress, and even deny what you have said to yourself just about as soon as you get out of the role of this or that interviewed character. This section helps you stay awake, to keep the reality of how amazing you are an undeniable reality.

It also provides a baseline post-test by which you may compare your initial understanding of your dream, as written in *associations*, with what you have learned from your journey. If your understanding about yourself, your dream or life drama, and your interviewed characters is different than it was in your initial written associations, then something has changed. What is it? Are your conclusions now the same as how you initially viewed your life issues? Are they different? Do they overlap? Is there a causal relationship, i.e., is the implication that your waking life issues will resolve themselves when you first address those issues of importance to your interviewed characters?

If you are like most students, you will be amazed at what you have learned. You may find yourself becoming somewhat addicted to the fascination that you have immediate access to such amazing acceptance, wisdom, compassion, and inner peace. You will want more, to know if all this is real or simply some sophisticated system of self-delusion.

"Some of the basic issues addressed by this group are"

Here are my initial associations to the dream:

> *My associations to this dream are* ... I really respect Ken Wilber and look forward not only to his next book, but am excited about the way he is influencing authorities in many different fields. For him to die in a car crash sounds like a warning that I am doing something to kill the part of myself which he represents – clear, objective, personally dedicated to transpersonal development and supporting others to do the same.

Here are basic issues addressed by Ken Wilber Dies:

- Don't take myself so seriously!
- When I screw up, don't waste time beating myself up.
- Practice thankfulness and appreciation in small ways.
- It's grandiose to feel so responsible or irresponsible!

When we compare where I started and where I was when I completed this process, I can see that this intrasocial group emphasized priorities that did not occur to me as I initially considered this dream.

Summary

- This section provides both a summary of your work and a post-test with which you can assess your growth through the process.
- Reviewing the summary section helps you stay awake; it helps you keep from falling back asleep.

Chapter 28

Evaluating your predictions

Application – the acid test of any yoga

Application is a powerful and essential part of the Dream Sociometric process. Its significance lies in its ability to move you beyond understanding to action, allowing you to prove or disprove for yourself the relevancy of your interview-elicited information without recourse to theory or dream experts. The claim is that by doing so you will both speed and simplify your growth into clarity, witnessing, increased wakefulness, the transpersonal, and into greater enlightenment. By making your life into an experimental laboratory, the understanding you have gained from your interviewed characters is translated into wisdom.

How can you tell what the "true meaning" of your dream is? By now you understand that you can't, because there is no one "true" meaning. The perspective of each and every interviewed character has its own validity. Like the blind men and the elephant, each perspective has a piece of the truth. Even after you combine all their perspectives and reach a conclusion, *that* perspective is only partial! The question of the meaning of a dream, has represented both the starting and end point of much dreamwork throughout history. To ask what is the meaning of a dream is to ask what the meaning of your life is. *The true test of the significance of any dream or waking drama is its usefulness in your life as a vehicle for your own transformation.* While those opinions offered by your interviewed characters could conceivably be considered to be the true meaning of the dream or life drama, you'll be settling for an endless multiplicity of meanings. IDL recommends that you do not search for *the* meaning of a dream, a life drama, or your life and instead start focusing on the awakenings that occur for you as you do more interviewing and work on applying the recommendations of various emerging potentials. Does your work with Dream Sociometry produce a more constructive lifestyle and a more satisfying life? Are you more or less accepting of yourself? Does your life more accurately, completely, and harmoniously reflect the priorities of your life compass?

You can tell how accurate your predictions are by looking at score totals in the Dream Sociomatrix or by evaluating the Dream Sociogram. In the case of the Dream Sociogram, look at the total scores in the right hand margin to find which character is most accepting. It will have the highest positive score. The least accepting will have the least positive score. If a character has a negative score, then the most negative score is the most rejecting as well as the least accepting. To find out which elements are most and least preferred, refer to the total scores at the bottom of the Dream Sociomatrix. Elements without dashes or asterisks in front of their names are characters. The highest positive score indicates the character most preferred by this intrasocial group as a whole. The character with either the lowest positive score or the highest negative score indicates the least preferred or the most rejected interviewed character. Determine the most and least preferred actions and feelings in the same way by evaluating those elements with dashes and asterisks.

The predictions for *Ken Wilber Dies* were:

Most Accepting:	Ken
Least Accepting:	Dream Self
Most Preferred Character:	Ken
Least Preferred Character:	Other Driver
Most Preferred Action:	none
Least Preferred Action:	killed
Most Preferred Emotion:	none
Least Preferred Emotion:	very upset

The actual preferences were:

Most Accepting:	Ken
Least Accepting:	Second Car
Most Preferred Character:	Ken
Least Preferred Character:	Other Driver
Most Preferred Action:	none
Least Preferred Action:	crash
Most Preferred Emotion:	none
Least Preferred Emotion:	very upset

I did better at these predictions than I usually do, probably because it is a small group of elements, and I have been at this for over 20 years. I generally score about 50%. Notice that while Dream Consciousness has the highest acceptance axis totals, it is not counted because it is not a dream element. Rather, it is defined as that consciousness that transcends and generates all possible dreams and forms. It generally is highly accepting because it is in the role of producer-director of the drama and personifying the perspective of causal witness.

Chapter 29

Using Dream Sociometry
with waking events

Is waking life a dream? Whether the answer is yes or no, waking life can certainly be approached *as if* it is a dream. Many people resist such a parallel, believing that it devalues life and creates a sense of detachment that is unhelpful and misleading. Others think that such an approach inevitably leads us to question our common assumptions about what is real, true and worth living and dying for. However, rather than devaluing consensus reality, life drama Dream Sociometric interviews increase the value of consensus reality. Because we make conscious decisions primarily in the waking state, IDL is finally assessed in terms of its usefulness to the ends and purposes of waking identity. The basic function of IDL is to create enlightenment, heightened wakefulness, lucidity, and clarity by aligning waking priorities, preferences, and perceptions with the priorities of life itself. The application of Dream Sociometry to waking events is another way to demonstrate that applicability as well as the dream-like nature of waking experience.

Dream Sociomatrices, Commentaries, and Dream Sociograms can be created around any waking issue or event: an argument, near-death experience, drug trip, meditation experience, romance, or rejection, or failure, resistance, humiliation, or abandonment. In creating a Dream Sociomatrix for a waking event, selected, key elements are listed in chronological order across the top of the Dream Sociomatrix and choosing characters are listed along the left margin, just as they would be for a dream. Interviewing and template construction proceed just as with a dream. Perhaps the most effective results occur when you use powerfully mythic events such as marriages, deaths, and other rites of passage, or accidents, traumas, or arguments. Socio-cultural events are even more likely to take on mythic proportions that clearly transcend self on a macrocosmic, transcultural scale, just as dreams clearly transcend self on a microcosmic, intrasocial scale.

The following example, 9/11, explores one of the pivotal events of the early 21st century. It was picked because at the time it had a palpably nightmarish quality to many, many people and contaminated ordinary waking life in intense and unusual ways for a period of time. It was as if a huge bell was rung, and you were standing right underneath it, or a huge tsunami came on shore, overwhelming everything in its path. Because most of us have strong associations to it, the hope is that this example will both clarify the process and motivate you to create your own on a life drama of your choice. There is no attempt made here to speak for others, although because this was a world dream the life issues and associations that came up reflected a world perspective rather than personal issues. Although I attempted to be in role throughout, you would create a different Dream Sociomatrix. However, deep listening connects us in a way in which one speaks for all. Your Dream Sociomatrix on 9/11 would speak for me. Some truths resonate, regardless of who speaks them.

Terrorists attack America

9/11/01
    Dillard (Created 09/19/01)
    (What if I had dreamed the horrifying actions of 9/11/01? How would IDL apply to such a dream? To work through this authentically, I must, to the best of my ability, treat the experience the nation and world are undergoing now as my dream and the issues that are confronting the world as my issues.) Here is that "dream," or better, nightmare:

> I am watching first one, then another huge jet full of passengers crash into the NYWTC in huge fireballs, then collapsing, killing thousands, including the terrorists. The Pentagon is also horribly attacked by a jet bomb. Fires rage. People are in shock, then grieving, then outraged. President Bush prepares the country for war.

Before you continue to read, answer the following questions:
    Of the following characters, which one do you think would be the most accepting of the others? Here are your choices:

> Dream Self (you in the dream)
> The New York Trade Center and Pentagon
> The Planes that were hijacked
> The Planes' passengers and victims in the towers and Pentagon
> The huge fireballs caused by the explosions
> The terrorists
> President Bush

Who do you think would be the least accepting? Who do you think would be the most preferred? Who do you think would be the least preferred?
    Of the following actions, which do you think would be the most preferred by this group? Which would be the least preferred?

> watching
> crash

collapse
killed
war

Of the following feelings, which do you think would be the most preferred by this group? Which would be the least preferred?

horrible
shock
grief
outrage

After you have read the following, compare your answers to the patterns of preference created by this particular intrasocial group.

My associations to this dream are . . . If I had this dream, I would wonder that I hate myself so much that I not only kill others but I kill myself. Why am I so angry at myself? I doubt that any compromise or resolution can come out of listening to these interviewed characters because the anger, suspicion, and distrust on both sides is so deep they just want to kill each other.

Three fundamental life issues

Formulate three questions, each addressing a different core life issue

- How do I create security for every part of myself, so that none of them want to repeat this?
- What is the appropriate response to take in the face of such a brutal, outrageous attack on myself and others?
- How do I learn to live in peace with all other parts of myself, even the ones I don't like or respect?

If I could resolve these issues, what difference would it make in my life?

As a global population, I would feel much more secure. Therefore, I would not be angry, and I might be able to trust and listen to other people that are different from me.

What do I think I need to do to be happy in my life?

Global population: "I want respect! I want my values, my beliefs, my way of life to be respected! You don't have to agree with me; you don't have to share my

Table 29.1

Dream Sociomatrix
Author: Dillard
Dream Date: 9/11/01
Name: Terrorists Attack America
SMX Date: 9/19/01

Choosers \ Chosen elements:	Dream Self-watching	NYTC	Pentagon	Planes	Victims	- Crash	*Fireballs	-Collapse	-Killed	Terrorist	*Horrible	*Shock	*Grief	*Outage	President Bush	- War	Character Raw Scores	Acceptance Axis Totals	Character Ambivalence
Dream Self	/2	2	2/2	2	2	/3	/3	/3	/3	/3	/3	/3	/3	/3	/1/2	/3	9/38	/29	
NYWTC/Pent.	/2	3	3	/3	2	/3	/3	/3	/3	/3	/3	/3	/3	/3	1	2	10/3	/24	M
Planes	/3	/1	/1	3	2	/3	/3	/3	/3	/3	/3	/3	/3	/3	1	2/2	8/37	/29	
Victims	/3	/1	/1	2/3	2	/3	/3	/3	/3	/3	/3	/3	/3	/3	1	2/2	7/40	/33	
Fireballs					1/1	3	3	/1		1	/3	/3	/3	/3			8/1	/9	
Terrorists	2	/3	/3	2	2	3	3	3	3	3	3	3	3	3	2	2	37/7	30	M
Pres. Bush	2	2	3	2	2	/3	/3	/3	/3	/3	/3	/3	/3	/3	1/1	1/1 2/2	12/30	/18	M
Dream Cons.					3	/3		/3	/3								3/9	/16	M
Raw Scores	3/10	7/5	8/7	11/6	13/1	6/18	6/15	3/19	3/18	4/15	3/15	3/15	3/15	3/15	5/3	10/9			
Axis Totals	/10	/7	2	1	5	12	/12	7	/16	/15	/11	/12	/12	/12	2	1			
ElementAmbi.	H	H	M		M	M	M								M	H			

© 1985 Joseph Dillard. All Rights Reserved.

beliefs. But respect my right to hold them! Respect the sacredness of my life if you want me to respect yours!"

Sociomatrix Scoring Key:

Blank = Don't Care; 1 = like; 2 = like a lot; 3 = love; /1 = dislike; /2 = dislike a lot; /3 = hate;

A(cceptance) = none of the above; two scores in one box indicate ambivalent feelings. (Underlined statements are extracted and placed below under "What I am saying to myself is . . .")

Dream Sociomatrix Commentary

"The reason I like, like (a lot, love, dislike, dislike a lot, hate, don't care about, or am non-attached toward) (dream element) is . . . " "What I liked/disliked most about being in this dream is . . ."

Dream Self: I really dislike myself a lot for letting this happen to me. How could I have been so blind? Why didn't I see this coming? I really don't like that I am watching because it feels so passive, so helpless! I feel so powerless just watching! The NYWTC is a living, breathing entity, home to thousands which I respect as a nurturing support for the lives of thousands and a powerful symbol of worldwide prosperity. It belongs to the world. When it was stabbed by that jet bomb I felt a huge part of myself die! I have mixed feelings about the Pentagon. I respect the people who work there as human beings. I understand the need for security within individuals, nations and the world. But this building is basically dedicated to threatening and killing people, if need be. So I have a love-hate relationship with power and intimidation.

I like the planes a lot because they provide an unimaginable degree of freedom. Technologically, they are miraculous. Although I knew none of the passengers personally, I care a great deal for the doomed passengers on these planes. My heart goes out to them in their needless deaths! I think of the terror many of them must have felt before they died. I hate the crash, the fireballs, the horrible collapses of the buildings. I feel great compassion for the thousands of helpless victims.

I hate the terrorists that they would do such a thing! I struggle to separate the human beings from their actions. I know that I am not actually hating the terrorists but their thoughts, actions and feelings. But it feels like I am hating the terrorists themselves because I am having trouble separating who they are from what they do, think and feel. I like President Bush because I respect the significance and importance of the role of president at a time like this. I don't like him a lot because I don't trust that he or his advisers have the vision to see past their anger and will simply create more terrorism through their reactivity. I don't understand how this war can be won. I think it is a war that everyone has to agree not to fight, because I see only losers in this war.

What I like most about being in this dream is nothing. What I dislike most about being in this dream is the feeling of powerlessness.

NYWTC/Pentagon: I am very, very, angry that you let me be attacked and destroyed! You deserve to be angry at yourself! You were neglectful and irresponsible, so complacent and lazy that you ignored not only my safety but ignored countless warnings that we were in danger! Your passivity is disgusting. Ignoring the injustices in the world won't make them go away. It just makes them bigger when they do finally happen. We hate these planes, although we understand that they were victims themselves. Still, they are the knives that stabbed us and killed us, in the case of WTC and wounded us badly, in the case of the Pentagon. While we feel sad for the passengers on the planes, we feel a lot worse for ourselves. We feel a lot like Dream Self does about this whole thing. We hate it and we hate what we are forced to feel. We like President Bush because we put a lot of hope in him to come through for us. But we really don't see how he can fix this situation, to right this wrong, much less keep it from happening again. War sounds like a good idea. What do we have to lose? We'll show people they can't treat us like this!

What I like most about being in this dream is nothing. Well, maybe if it wakes Dream Self up to the fact that we need a whole lot more defending than we're getting, that's something that's important. What I dislike most about being in this dream is getting destroyed and feeling pretty hopeless about stopping it.

Planes: We hate Dream Self for being so passive and not taking care of us. He wants the power and the freedom we give him but he is unwilling to exercise the responsibility that we require. He is like a baby playing with matches around gasoline! He's just blown up his house and charred himself! We dislike the WTC and the Pentagon because they killed us when we slammed into them. But we can't dislike them too much, because they were just sitting there. They were helpless victims like we are. Still, if they hadn't been in our way, they wouldn't have killed us. We love ourselves! We are big, beautiful and extraordinarily sophisticated! We like our passengers a lot. Our job is to serve them. We are so in touch with our own death and the deaths of our passengers that we really just can't care about the thousands who died when we slammed into these buildings. We hate that they died, though. We hate those terrorists! There's nothing that President Bush can do that can make a difference for us now, anyway. Maybe he can do something to make our brothers safer, but I doubt it. I think a lot of steps can be taken that create an illusion of security, but maybe none of us have ever really been safe. Maybe that was an illusion. Maybe none of us will ever really be safe. We feel neutral about Bush, because we think he's basically impotent. But if he can set a positive tone of responsibility and mutual respect, perhaps things can get better. We like the idea of going to war a lot because the terrorists deserve to be punished. But we also dislike the idea of going to war a lot because we think it will just hurt the innocent, mostly, inflame passions and drain resources that could better be spent defusing the causes of terrorism.

What I like most about being in this dream is nothing. What I dislike most about being in this dream is being a helpless victim and the means to the destruction of thousands.

Passengers/Victims: We feel like the planes do, since they are victims just like we are. But while they love themselves and we do like them a lot, we also hate them because they are the instruments of our death! So we have a lot of mixed feelings about them. We like ourselves a lot. How could we have known that this would happen to us??? Maybe we should care about all those victims, but we are so tied up in the horror, grief and anger we feel about our own deaths that we don't have the energy to feel much empathy or even sympathy. We hate that they were murdered! We hate those terrorists! We have to hope that President Bush can create a vision for the country that sees beyond reprisals and a mere escalation of the round of violence. We have to hope that he will foster ways to reduce those factors that inflame the passions of terrorists. Basically, we agree mostly with the Planes.

What I like most about being in this dream is nothing. I hate it. What I dislike most about being in this dream is feeling that our deaths are for nothing

Fireballs: I don't care about Dream Self or that he is watching. Well, I guess I like that he is a witness to my raw, uncontrollable power. I don't care about the NYWTC or the Pentagon at all, except that they become fuel for me to exalt myself in my glory. The planes and passengers are fuel. The crash allows me to live, so I love it. I love myself! I love to burn! The collapse basically puts me out, so I don't like that. Whether people die or not, whether things get destroyed or not, is no concern of mine. The terrorists allowed me to express myself, to make my glorious nature known to all. So I like them. Other than living fully, I really don't care. What I like most about being in this dream is being free, powerful and fully alive!! What I dislike most about being in this dream is that it had to end. I would have liked to have burned forever.

Terrorists: We have only contempt for Dream Self. He is not worth hating or even disliking. We like a lot that he is watching, because he is learning of his powerlessness against us, his complacency. He is dreaming his dream of safety and security while he parasitically lives off of us, robbing our lands of their resources, occupying our holy places, supporting those who commit terrorist acts against our women and children. If we have to die, he will die too. But in our deaths the glory and superiority of Islam will shine. They are sleeping cowards; we are courageous holy warriors who put our faith above our comfort and our lives, so unlike what these swine do. Our deaths, the deaths of these symbols of American arrogance, the deaths of all these accomplices to the murder of our cultures, bring glory to us and our cause.

We hate these buildings for what they symbolize – the arrogant attempt to dominate our land, our culture, our faith. The planes we like a lot as instruments of our punishment. We like the passengers because we can make a greater statement through their terror and helpless deaths. We dislike them as American taxpayers who support the abuse of our culture. We love the carnage, horror, grief and even the outrage, because now they know exactly how we feel and we have felt for decades now, humiliated by their arrogance and conceit. What we like most about being in this dream is waking Dream Self and America up to us. Making them realize that they not only cannot ignore us, that they can't just take us seriously. By our deaths we are forcing them to recognize, address and respect our legitimate needs. So our deaths are good. War is good, because we will triumph. The deaths of all these people is absolutely necessary. What I dislike most about being in this dream is nothing.

Bush: I pretty much feel like Dream Self. I put on a brave face, but deep down I don't know if I have what it takes to handle this one. I very much want to go to war, because it gives me an agenda around which I can unite the people. I was going to have trouble otherwise. But I just don't know about this war. I want to get revenge, but I am not sure who to attack and I don't see an exit strategy. I feel pretty uneasy about this. . . . What I like most about being in this dream is having a chance to give hope and prove that I'm a capable leader. What I dislike most about being in this dream is that I'm out of my depth. What I dislike is that I really don't know what to do and that this is going to make me look powerless and incapable if I'm not careful.

Dream Consciousness: I really hated having to create this drama. I hate that Dream Self was so fast asleep, so complacent, that I had to kick him hard in the ass to wake him up. I had to not just make him mad, but angry. It's a risk I'm taking, because he could use his anger to turn me off. He could use his anger to hurt himself. But if I don't wake him up, he'll fall even deeper asleep. Then I will have to kick him even harder to wake him up. So now I've hurt him. But I've got his attention. Now that he's alert, is he going to listen, or just stay angry? I hate that I have been forced to hurt my own creations. But it is time to wake up or die. If he does not wake up, then what good am I? Death is better than the selfish insolence of somnambulism.

What I like most about creating this dream is my willingness to take great risks in order to create a greater good. My hope is that Joseph will come to respect the needs of ALL parts of himself instead of wasting his life ignoring the legitimate needs of parts of himself and therefore at war with himself. What I dislike most about creating this dream is the pain, fear and anger it has caused.

What surprises me about what I've heard is . . . The planes said that safety had been an illusion, that they never really had been safe and that their brothers never really would be. This made me think about living with insecurity instead of pretending to be safe, to live with the knowledge that there is nobody or no thing that can guarantee that I won't die horribly tomorrow. It causes me to think about what it would be like to live happily in that knowledge. Is it possible? If I do it, I won't have unrealistic expectations of the President, or the government, or of airplanes that they will protect or support me. I won't put my confidence, faith, or trust in people or things that are fundamentally unreliable. That's hard to do, because I get used to thinking that they are reliable and will support me. Then I blame them when I get reminded that this is basically a false trust. Still, I pay taxes with the expectation that I will get something back. Maybe I am paying to reduce the odds that bad things will happen, but I am not buying an insurance policy that bad things won't happen to me.

Sounds to me like I am being forced to move, as a social being, into a radical existentialism in which I have no "thing" or person that I can base my happiness or security on. I have to learn to live with radical meaninglessness and anxiety and still be happy. I do it on a personal level. Can I do it on a social level?

I am also surprised that the passengers and victims dislike most that their deaths are for nothing. It makes me want their deaths to inspire not war, but a real dialogue that can result in the protection of the rights of people everywhere so that this can never happen again. If that happened, then they would not have died in vain.

I realized while the Terrorists were talking that "Dream Self" is mostly the voice of America in this dream, a character which was not included in the narrative.

Dream Consciousness is not beyond having feelings. In fact, it has very strong feelings about a few things and none at all about the others. This is because it sees much of this "dream" as a necessary drama from which it is detached, but it feels for the pain it has caused the actors, for whom the drama is real.

Dream Summary Commentary

("What part of this dreamer's consciousness do you personify? "The reason why I am in this dream is . . . " and, "This intrasocial group came together to . . . ")

NYWTC/Pentagon: I most closely personify your pride in your public image as the best, the brightest, the strongest. I also personify your world presence and your dominating power economically and militarily. The reason why I am in this dream is to make you question your unquestioned superiority and your ability to get your way irrespective of the needs and wishes of others. You believe too much in your persona, your ego. This intrasocial group came together to wake you up, to humble you, to teach you not to base your value or your existence on us, because we are transient and will not always be there for you.

Planes: I most closely personify your freedom and sense of security as you expand in whatever direction you want to go in life. The reason why I am in this dream is to force you to understand that as long as you ignore or repress the freedom and security of any aspect of yourself, you can never really be free or secure. This intrasocial group came together to force you to listen to your larger self and its' needs.

Passengers/Victims: I most closely personify the parts of you that get victimized when you ignore the needs of your larger self. The reason why I am in this dream is to cause you to recognize the pain you are causing yourself. This intrasocial group came together to motivate you to deeply listen to yourself.

Fireballs: I most closely personify your power run amok. The more you develop, the more freedom and power you have. If you do not grow in responsibility and cooperation at the same time, the imbalance between these two will cause your power to explode and destroy you. You cannot grow at the expense of perspectives forever and remain secure. The reason why I am in this dream is to force you to rectify this balance by understanding just how capable of destroying yourself you are. This intrasocial group came together to create anger and fear to generate motivation for deep listening to hurting emerging potentials.

Terrorists: I most closely personify the disenfranchised, ignored, abused, humiliated emerging potentials that are courageous, proud and demanding of respect at any cost. We are parts of you that would rather kill you and us too than live like dogs under your rule. The reason why I am in this dream is to scare you awake and to force you to feel our pain. This intrasocial group came together to give you a wake-up call. If you respond with more repression, we will kill you. We are not afraid to die. Are you?

Bush: I most closely personify the executive function that is so closely identified with preserving appearances and the status quo that it favors repression over dialogue and compromise. The reason why I am in this dream is to remind you that if you keep thinking about your problems in the same way you have in the past – strengthen yourself, repress your enemies – that eventually your own power will destroy you. This intrasocial group came together to get you to put your faith in yourself rather than your government or your personality or your public image.

Dream Consciousness: I most closely personify the world-patterning consciousness that created this socio-political drama. The reason why I created this dream is to help you to understand that you are at war with yourself and repression will only make it worse. You have to listen to yourself or you will kill yourself. This intrasocial group came together to enact this dilemma in a way you cannot ignore, repress, or avoid dealing with.

Dream Commentary

> "If I could change this dream in any way, would I change it? If so, how?"

NYWTC/Pentagon: It wouldn't ever happen! The terrorists would be caught before they boarded the plane or overwhelmed by the passengers or they would have a change of heart! But if it did happen, then the damage would be minimal. But if we were destroyed, like in the dream, then I suppose the way I would change this dream would be for our deaths to not be in vain. I would want a more secure, mutually respectful world to be the heritage of our deaths.

Planes: Yes.

Passengers/Victims: We have to go through the stages of dealing with grief. But once we have accepted the reality of our deaths, we need to expand that acceptance to all others. Because after we die, nothing matters. Being right doesn't matter. Being American doesn't matter. Being strong doesn't matter, because we're still dead. The only thing that can make a difference, from our point of view, is acceptance. Accept that we are dead, accept each other. And out of that acceptance will come mutual respect and out of that mutual respect will come a security based on that which doesn't die instead of bombs and buildings.

Fireballs: I like this dream the way it is! I get to play and I get noticed!

Terrorists: We need to do this in order to get noticed and our grievances taken seriously. We have no confidence that you will get it short of our inflicting pain and suffering on you. In fact, we fear that you will forget this and go back to your comfortable, self-indulgent ways.

Bush: Give me the strength to set an example of good listening, not just to the points of view I agree with, but to the needs of those who terrorize us. Then give me the vision to embrace responses that respect the legitimate concerns of those parts of myself that hate me.

Dream Consciousness: This dream, as gruesome as it is, needs to happen. You are listening to its members, allowing disagreements and hurts to be aired. This dream is serving its purpose. I would recommend that a "cabinet meeting" of these characters be convened in which all viewpoints are heard and a genuine attempt is made to address the needs and legitimate interests of all parties.

Does anyone object?

No! We all are willing to discuss where to from here.

NYWTC/Pentagon, Planes, Passengers/Victims, Bush: We demand justice and compensation.

Terrorists: We demand that you get your military out of the Middle East. You defile our holy sites. We demand you stop financially and militarily supporting Israel because it is a terrorist state that kills our wives and children. We demand that you get Israel to stop attacking us.

NYWTC/Pentagon, Planes, Passengers/Victims, Bush: If we were able and willing to give you what you want, would that not validate the effectiveness of terrorism? Would that not be appeasement? And even if it didn't, could you be trusted to bring to justice those who have committed these crimes against humanity? Could you be trusted to compensate us for our losses which are so huge there is no possible compensation that would be sufficient?

Terrorists: Don't trust us. Empower an international force to keep all warring parties apart. As long as we are represented in that force, we will accept it. It will guarantee your security.

NYWTC/Pentagon, Planes, Passengers/Victims, Bush: You must turn the perpetrators over to the International Court of Justice in The Hague. We do not trust Islamic courts.

Terrorists: We will compensate you with our oil revenues if your military leaves our countries, an international force protects Palestinians from the Israelis and you stop supporting Israel financially and militarily.

NYWTC/Pentagon, Planes, Passengers/Victims, Bush: We are unwilling to stop supporting Israel, but we may consider equal support for the Palestinians.

Terrorists: You will not need to support Israel if an international military force is guaranteeing its' safety.

NYWTC/Pentagon, Planes, Passengers/Victims, Bush: In order to pull out of the middle east, we must no longer be dependent on your oil for our economic security.

Terrorists: If you can get to the Moon, surely you can learn to be independent in oil!

NYWTC/Pentagon, Planes, Passengers/Victims, Bush: You don't understand. There are a lot of powerful people in our country who would go broke if our economy was not based on your oil.

Terrorists: Becoming energy-self-sufficient would increase your national security much more than fighting with us will ever do. Would you rather fight with us or regenerate your economy by developing alternative renewable sources of energy?

NYWTC/Pentagon, Planes, Passengers/Victims, Bush: Why are you telling us this? You will go broke without our money!

Terrorists: We would rather have our heritage and our culture than your money. The corrupt ruling classes are the ones that want you to stay dependent on our oil – not us. NYWTC/Pentagon, Planes, Passengers/Victims, Bush: We have the outlines of a possible agreement here. If we get the UN to impose a cease-fire between Israel and the Palestinians, with armed troops on the ground, if we agree to remove our air stations from Saudi Arabia and if we agree to compensate Palestine with yearly appropriations equal to those we give Israel, what do we get in return?

Terrorists: We will hand over whomever you think is guilty to The Hague and abide by the decision of the court. We will abide by international judgments as to what is fair and reasonable compensation for our terrorist acts, as long as you get Israel to agree to do the same for its terrorism against us. We will preach against terrorism and forbid it. We will continue to hold ourselves liable for any terrorist acts and agree to hand over any terrorists to an international tribunal.

(All of the above negotiation requires interpretation on a personal level: basically, parts of identity require justice and compensation from other parts. What does this mean? How could that be done? On an intrapersonal level that basically means respect and non-interference, if not actual assistance at meeting ends that are desired by the aggrieved parts of self. Other parts feel violated and imposed upon. They demand to be left alone. This is as if there are parts of ourselves that are natural that want to stay that way or parts of ourselves who value their way of looking at the world, even if it is very different from what we, as waking identities, accept. It would be as if interviewed characters were demanding that waking identity stop controlling them through lucid dream manipulation or, more indirectly, through indulging some harmful addiction such as alcohol or sex. It could also be consistent abusive self-talk that discounts the worth of aspects of ourselves.)

Dreamage

(A rewrite of the dream based on a consensus of interviewed character recommendations. If there is no consensus, there can be no dreamage. A synthesis group dream is usually its own dreamage. Read it over before sleep as an affirmation of a higher pattern of internal integration and healing.)

There was no agreement on a dreamage.

Waking Commentary

("Character,) If you were in charge of my life today, would you change it? If so, how? How would you handle my three fundamental life issues?")

NYWTC/Pentagon: In light of our previous negotiation, I would share power. I would listen more. I would compromise with other parts of myself a lot more.

Planes: I would not live my life assuming that I am free and secure. I wouldn't take those things for granted. I would constantly be checking with other parts of myself that have the ability to destroy me or see if *they* feel free and secure.

Passengers/Victims: I would not go through my life assuming that I was safe and deserving. I would change my expectations to take into consideration the needs of others a lot more than I have been doing.

Fireballs: I'm OK with being contained and you can trust me to explode if you give me a chance!

Terrorists: If you listen to us we will be less angry and less likely to strike out.

Bush: I have got to realize that my constituency is more than just the parts of myself that I like or that I feel loyal to. I have got to represent the needs of *everyone*.

Dream Consciousness: You're getting it!

Life Issue Commentary

(Is there a life issue which you would like to ask these interviewed characters about? "
Life Issue: Deeper, longer, more regular meditation.
("If I were this dreamer, this is how I would handle this life issue:")

NYWTC/Pentagon: I would just surrender, since I'm dead. There would be no resistance, including interfering thoughts and feelings.

Planes: I would work at staying above the problems of the day, the concerns of everyday life.

Passengers/Victims: I would not trust in my agenda or in my daily routines to get me through, because they are fundamentally undependable.

Fireballs: We don't burn without oxygen. Meditate high up in the atmosphere and in space and I can't burn.

Terrorists: Do IDL to listen to the emerging potentials. It will defuse resistance to equanimity, evoke compassion and awaken wisdom.

Bush: The country runs itself. I need to inspire, then get out of the way. Dream consciousness: Identify with me when you meditate.

Point of maximum leverage

> *("Of all the above recommendations for daily change, if there was one in particular that you would strongly recommend that the dreamer specifically apply during the coming week, in order to make maximum progress, what would it be?")*

NYWTC/Pentagon: Meditate. Planes: Meditate Passengers/Victims: Meditate. Fireballs:

> Terrorists: Listen to the disenfranchised within yourself. Bush: Meditate. Dream consciousness: Meditate.

Action Plan

(All of these recommendations for waking life applications are not necessarily helpful or of equal importance. You have to decide how you wish to prioritize them and what you want to do with them. But take some action! It is a way of demonstrating that you take your inner direction seriously. If you have it wrong, future intrasocial groups will cybernetically correct your course.)

- Meditate.
- When meditating, become Dream Consciousness.
- Do IDL to deeply listen to and move toward consensus with aspects of yourself.

Action Plan Pre-Sleep Rehearsal

(Imagine you are going about your day tomorrow. See yourself dealing with your life issues in the ways recommended by your interviewed characters. Write this image out as a pre-sleep suggestion. Read it over several times before going to sleep.)

I am sitting around a large table at the UN in Manhattan. It's the Security Council. The other interviewed characters from this dream are in the other chairs. We are negotiating out our disagreements, as above. Now we are meditating. I am experiencing myself as Dream Consciousness.

"What I am saying to myself is"

(A rewording of key comments of interviewed characters as statements that you are making about yourself.)

- I really dislike myself a lot for letting this happen to me.
- What I dislike most . . . is the feeling of powerlessness.
- I deserve to be angry at myself.
- I am neglectful and irresponsible, so complacent and lazy that I ignore not only my safety but ignore countless warnings that I am in danger!
- War sounds like a good idea. What do I have to lose? I'll show myself I can't treat myself like this!
- I need to be woken up to the fact that parts of myself need a whole lot more defending than they are getting.
- I want the power and the freedom prosperity gives me, but I am unwilling to exercise the responsibility that it requires.
- I am not worth hating or even disliking.
- My death is good. War is good, because I will triumph. The deaths of all these parts of myself is absolutely necessary.
- I don't know if I have what it takes to handle this one.
- I very much want to go to war with myself, because it gives me an agenda around which I can unite myself.
- I really don't know what to do and that this is going to make me look powerless and incapable if I'm not careful.

Some of the basic issues addressed by this intrasocial group are:

- I am torn between fighting to express control and confidence and to act out my rage in a self-righteous crusade for justice on the one hand and doing the much harder work of examining how I brought this on myself and deeply listening to the legitimate concerns of other, disowned, parts of myself.
- How I am much more like the disowned terrorist within me than I recognize or begin to admit.
- How my self-criticism neutralizes and therefore cuts me off from higher sources of guidance and grace. (As seen by the neutralization of Dream Consciousness in its Sociogram placement.)
- How strong preferences tend to create reactive, equally strong oppositional strong preferences within me.

At this point, what is your understanding of what you think you need to do to be happy in your life?

Meditate a lot more and do IDL regularly so that I can become aware of and defuse my internal conflicts before they get to this point.

Sociogram scoring key

To determine placement, find the appropriate axis and count one degree of preference for each concentric circle, starting at the center, which is zero.

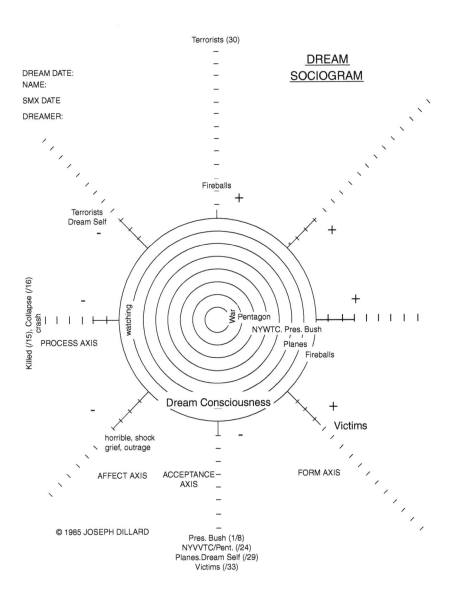

Terrorists (30)

DREAM
SOCIOGRAM

DREAM DATE:
NAME:
SMX DATE
DREAMER:

Fireballs

Terrorists
Dream Self

Killed (/15), Collapse (/16)
crash

PROCESS AXIS

watching

War   Pentagon
NYWTC. Pres. Bush
Planes
Fireballs

Dream Consciousness

Victims

horrible, shock
grief, outrage

AFFECT AXIS   ACCEPTANCE—
AXIS

FORM AXIS

© 1985 JOSEPH DILLARD

Pres. Bush (1/8)
NYVVTC/Pent. (/24)
Planes.Dream Self (/29)
Victims (/33)

Positive scores are placed on "+" axes and indicate degree of preference. Negative scores are placed on "-" axes and indicate degree of rejection. Vertical (acceptance axis) scores (choosing characters) are taken from the right end of the Sociomatrix. This indicates how accepting or rejecting "choosers" are. Element (chosen characters, actions, and feelings) are taken from the bottom of the Sociomatrix. This indicates how preferred or rejected chosen elements are.

Sociogram Commentary

Overall Pattern: This is a nightmare Dream Sociogram, as destructive interviewed characters are placed on the positive pole of the acceptance axis while nurturing or victimized interviewed characters are relegated to the negative or rejecting pole of that axis. This indicates not only extreme self-loathing but extreme powerlessness.

Acceptance Axis: The terrorists are the self-aspect that have control and power in this intrasocial group, even though they are far outnumbered by the positive, neutral, or victimized interviewed characters. We have a very extreme polarization, moving from +28 to -29. This is a 57-point preferential swing, indicating an amazing degree of internal polarization. While Dream Consciousness is not only relatively neutral, but neutralized as well. It too had extremely strong positive and negative preferences, indicating that it also was emotionally invested in this intrasocial group in contradictory ways, as validated by its remarks. It is powerless to do anything other than depict the causative karmic patterns externally (in dreams and in waking life) in the hope that someone will stop, listen, and see.

Form Axis: The Passengers/Victims are the most preferred interviewed characters. The big surprise here comes on the negative pole of this axis: Dream Self is viewed by this group as a surrogate of the hated antagonist, the Terrorists. This is very different from how Dream Self sees himself in the dream, although he dislikes himself a lot as well. This pairing of Dream Self with the Terrorists in the preferences of the group as a whole is a statement of Dream Self's (disowned) responsibility for creating and maintaining this pattern of self-abuse. Dream Self is seen by this intrasocial group as a whole to be in opposition to the victimized aspects of self, and it is a strong opposition (-11 to +13, 24 degrees of preference, a lot for the form axis).

Process Axis: Another unusual and fairly astonishing feature of this particular intrasocial group is the complete absence of *any* preferred actions on the process axis. There are absolutely no preferred behaviors for this intrasocial group. This is extremely unusual. It is ironic that a behavior that would normally be expected to be highly rejected, "war," is the *least* rejected by this intrasocial group. This implies that this group is strongly disposed to conflict going forward, although it does not prefer it.

Affect Axis: There are no redeeming positive emotions in this intrasocial group, although there were any number of positive preferences expressed by many interviewed characters, demonstrating that there was much identification with strong feelings, many of which tend to create their opposite.

Dream Group Dynamics Commentary

> (*In which the various interviewed characters are provided with an opportunity to express their thoughts on their relationships with their fellow interviewed characters.*)

NYWTC/Pentagon: I don't have the power to change this intrasocial group. Planes: If we listen to each other, perhaps we can find some way forward. Passengers/Victims: I am willing to listen if I can be heard.
Fireballs: I am pleased with the status quo.

Terrorists: I am in no mood to listen to any of you. I have demands that have to be met or I'll kill us all.

Bush: We have no choice. They are like a cancer. We can't love it to death. It's time for surgery.

Dream Consciousness: There is no grace in this intrasocial group. It will have to come from a combination of meditation and continuing dialogue. This is a start.

In summary

Based on the patterns seen in the Dream Sociogram, the perspective of Americans is at least as much responsible for terrorism as are the terrorists themselves. In addition, it can be predicted, based on the relationships of this intrasocial group, that war is the most likely course of action going forward. It can also be predicted that war is unlikely to resolve this problem, because it is not a behavior which will change the preference relationships between the various interviewed characters.

The Fireball is a totally powerful, amoral part of myself.

This is a bleak pattern. No one is really in a mood to listen to the needs of anyone else because they fear that would be a sign of appeasement and capitulation that would simply inspire more abuse. It is not realistic to expect change to come from any source but Dream Self, who has to demonstrate leadership to everyone, including Bush, on this, by insisting on continuing dialogue and attunement to a transcendent pattern of healing through meditation.

We can see from the above example that *any* life event can potentially be treated as a dream. If we so choose, we can create Dream Sociomatrices about any conceivable waking event. When we do so, we find that the distinction between dreaming and waking experience is mostly an artifice of waking identity. It is not that waking is therefore illusory or that dreaming is therefore real; it is that our reality judgments are seen to be tools, not safe harbors or absolutes upon which to base our sense of self. IDL can now be properly understood as a transpersonal technology that uses any and all form, regardless of the state of consciousness in which it manifests, as a vehicle for transformation.

Appendix I
Ken Wilber dies commentaries

This example of Dream Sociometry is used to explain how to create a Dream Sociomatrix and Dream Sociogram in the text, *Dream Sociometry*. It was chosen for several reasons. Because it is nightmarish, it provides an example of how Dream Sociometry and IDL addresses nightmares. It is short, with not so many elements, and, therefore, is a relatively simple and straightforward example to demonstrate Dream Sociomatrix and Dream Sociogram construction. The title involves a well-known figure in integral circles, which ties into the collective or common heritage of both dreams and waking life issues. The title is also provocative, raising questions like, "Is this precognitive?" (No.) "Does the author have some sort of love-hate relationship with Wilber?" (No.)

Ken Wilber Dies
08/27/01
Joseph Dillard

I hear that Ken Wilber and his girlfriend are killed in a head-on car crash. I am very upset.

My associations to this dream are . . . I really respect Ken Wilber and look forward not only to his next book, but am excited about the way he is influencing authorities in many different fields. For him to die in a car crash sounds like a warning that I am doing something to kill the part of myself which he represents – clear, objective, personally dedicated to spiritual development and supporting others to do the same.

What are three life issues you are currently dealing with in your life?

- How am I killing the part of myself that is like Ken Wilber?
- How can I improve my meditation?
- How can I discipline myself to lose this last 15 pounds?

If I could resolve these issues, what difference would it make in my life?

I could help more people understand how they sabotage their spiritual development and what they can do to stop it.

I could help more people meditate better. I would feel less hypocritical and more authentic about practicing what I'm preaching.

I could help other people stick to and attain challenging personal goals. It would increase my self-esteem and get one more irritation out of my life.

What do I think I need to do to be happy in my life?

Listen to myself and demonstrate that I respect myself by acting on the good I hear by making changes in my waking life; give others, especially those who I have the most trouble with, the love and respect I desire.

Sociomatrix Scoring Key

Blank = Don't Care; 1 = like; 2 = like a lot; 3 = love; /1 = dislike; /2 = dislike a lot; /3 = hate;

A(cceptance) = none of the above; two scores in one box indicate ambivalent feelings.

Sociomatrix Commentary

"The reason I like, like (a lot, love, dislike, dislike a lot, hate, don't care about, or am non-attached toward) (dream element) is . . ." "What I liked/disliked most about being in this dream is . . ."

Dream Self: I like myself a lot because I respect the integrity of my life and my efforts to live in balance and teach others to do so. I love Ken Wilber because I see him doing the same and being much more successful at it than I am. I like his girlfriend because she is meaningful to him; I really don't know much about her except the little I've read about her in *One Taste*. I have no feelings one way or the other about the cars. He is probably driving and it's probably a jeep. The other car seems to be a new model in good shape as well. I hate that there is a head-on crash, that they are killed and that I am very upset. I want to dislike the other driver a lot and blame him for the crash, but I don't know if that is accurate or not. What I like most about being in this dream is nothing. I feel like I'm not in it, but a spectator who

gets the news. What I dislike most about being in this dream is
the sense of tragedy and loss that I feel.

Ken Wilber: I love Joseph for his dedication and out of my desire that he, as
well as many others, carry on my work, now that I can't. I love
myself because I have lived my life in a way that has reflected my
ideals to the best of my ability. I love my girlfriend very much and
really hate that she died too. I like my car and feel terrible that it's
now destroyed. The second car I have no feelings about. I hate the
needless waste of this head-on collision. It was unnecessary and
entirely avoidable. I hate it that I have to die unnecessarily and for
no good purpose. I like a lot that Joseph is very upset. He should
be. I dislike the other driver because he caused this wreck! What
I like most about being in this dream is nothing! What I dislike
most about being in this dream is getting killed for no good reason or purpose. It's so futile!

Girlfriend: I really appreciate Joseph's concern. I love Ken very much! I like
myself a lot and feel really bad that I am dead. It feels so needless
and meaningless. I don't like that other car a lot because it killed
us, which I hate. I like a lot that Joseph is very upset; he should be!
The other driver was thoughtless. His negligence not only ended
his life but ours too! What I like most about being in this dream
is being recalled so that I can now express my anger about being
killed needlessly! What I dislike most about being in this dream
is losing Ken and losing my life, all out of thoughtless, brain dead,
mindless, sleepwalking through life on the part of the other driver.
He swerved in front of us!

Car: I feel pretty much like everybody else so far, except that I like
myself a lot and really hate that I had a head on crash. I feel that
I didn't do my job and let Ken and his girlfriend down, although
I can't see how I could have done anything differently. I hate the
other driver! What I like most about being in this dream is having
a chance to express how much I hate this!! What I dislike most
about being in this dream is playing the victim. I know I'm not
really dead, because I'm talking right now, but I don't have the
same physical reality that I would have if I had continued to live
in that dream!

Second Car: I don't know any of these people but I feel terrible that I killed
them! I guess they were pretty special and now they're gone! I am
pretty upset too because I was alive, doing my job and now I'm
gone and I can't! My driver was thoughtless and inconsiderate.
I don't like him at all! What I like most about being in this dream
is that I have the opportunity to express myself by being recalled
and listened to. What I dislike most about being in this dream is
that *I am the instrument by which insensitivity and injustice occurs.*

Other Driver:	I pretty much agree with everyone else. I WAS to blame! I was thoughtless, insensitive and careless. I hate it that I killed these people and myself. Dream Self has every right to be upset with me! I am upset with myself very much! I hate myself for what I did! What I like most about being in this dream is nothing. What I dislike most about being in this dream is being responsible for all this needless tragedy!
Dream Consciousness:	I love all these characters that I created. I am sorry that they are so upset! It's really not necessary! What I want them to do is see beyond their expectations and be thankful in all circumstances, even those that seem unfair and unjust. What I like most about creating this dream is demonstrating how even great tragedy can be seen in a broader context devoid of drama. What I dislike most about creating this dream is that I had to go to these lengths to get Joseph's attention to teach him this truth. If he would just accept it and practice it, I wouldn't have to scare him to get his attention!

What surprises me about what I've heard is

I notice that I care about another character more strongly than I do about myself. I also notice that I have very strong negative preferences, which doesn't feel particularly enlightened! It is curious to me that I have no concern for the driver of the other car. I don't even include him as a character, although I should! I will go back and add him in.

Ken Wilber appears to more or less be a surrogate because his preferences are pretty much the same as mine. The exception is that he likes a lot that I am very upset, which makes sense, from his perspective, but the preference ends up being opposite that of Dream Self. He provides new information – that the crash was indeed an accident and that it was caused by the other driver.

The girlfriend is also a surrogate of the dreamer because her preferences are very similar, but even a bit harder, more polarized because she dislikes the second car, where Dream Self does not. I don't think I've ever had a character say that what it liked most about being in a dream was "being recalled" so that the character could express its feelings! She states that the other driver swerved in front of them.

This reminds me of some thoughts that I had yesterday or the day before as I was driving. I was thinking about teaching (my daughter) Kira how to drive (she's thirteen) and about how I wanted to teach her to pray for other drivers, about how any of them at any time could swerve in front of her or pull out in front of her, about how we drive taking for granted that other drivers are going to do what they need to do to keep us safe, but in fact our lives are always in the hands of oncoming drivers and any one of them could change the course of our lives forever. So I started praying for the other drivers and thought about how doing so changes the consciousness of the cells of my body, especially the water, which makes up 90+ % of my body. I imagined those cells transformed into perfect patterns of thankfulness and appreciation.

The car is ambivalent toward itself, liking itself but disliking itself for "letting Ken and his girlfriend down."

The remarks of the second car remind me of my recent loss of my father and before that, my mother. They were pretty special and now they're gone. I am surprised that the second car, which is blamed in part for the wreck, is also angry and blaming its driver, because it is dead too!

The awareness of all these characters that they are not "really" dead because they still can express their feelings contradicts their anger at having their paths disrupted. Do they have reason to be really upset or not? Are they dead or not? It would seem that they are not and that therefore they are all overreacting at the fact that their path has been interrupted and therefore their live path has not lived up to their expectations. It sounds like the crash isn't the problem, but their expectations that the crash was unfair is the problem!

Other Driver is a part of myself that thinks it is itself bad because it does stupid, tragic, thoughtless things. Because it makes bad choices, it punishes itself. The thought that comes to my mind is "How much do I need to beat up on myself when I kill the best parts of myself? How long do I need to blame myself or stay on a guilt trip when I slip up and destroy the best parts of myself? Is it really helpful? Does it really change anything? I also realize that in so doing I am not distinguishing between who I am and what I do. I am not "loving the actor but hating the action." After all, this IS a dream! We, Dream Self and the various characters in the dream, could all learn from our experience, laugh about the intensity of our feelings and get on with our lives.

I need to practice being thankful in all situations, just as I was reminding myself and practicing as I was driving the other day. This dream came to strongly reinforce that practice and that perspective. I need not waste time beating myself up when I screw up!

Such conclusions reflect the practical applications that can result from putting both dream and life dramas in perspective. Notice that Dream Sociometry merges dream and life dramas. From the perspective of life, there is no difference, because each is the mirror of the other and by awakening within one you awaken within the other.

The Dream Summary Commentary

("What part of this dreamer's consciousness do you personify? The reason why I am in this dream and this dream group came together is . . .")

Ken Wilber: I most closely personify the parts of Joseph that he admires and respects the most, the parts that are dedicated to service but which balance it with a healthy dedication to balancing body, mind and life in his own life. The reason why I am in this dream is to help him let go of his expectations that he grow into me, to feel OK about who he is right now and where he is right now. Life is always going to be an interrupted journey. This intrasocial group came together to teach moment to moment non-attachment, thankfulness and appreciation.

Girlfriend: I most closely personify the more emotionally attached, caring part of Joseph. I hate not being able to be supportive, because that's how I justify my existence! The reason why I am in this dream is to let go of the need to do that. This intrasocial group came together to help Joseph understand, through working through it, that life goes on, even when it doesn't live up to his expectations. Therefore, he needs to drop his unrealistic expectations and his guilt when he doesn't live up to them.

Car: I most closely personify Joseph's body. The reason why I am in this dream is to help him let go of his fear of physical death so that he can live more courageously as he grows older. This intrasocial group came together to teach love in all circumstances, even the most painful ones.

Second Car: I most closely personify the parts of your physical life that are self- destructive and end up even destroying itself, such as bad eating habits or out-of-control genes that cause your body to break down regardless of what you do. The reason why I am in this dream is to help you to learn compassion toward your own self-destruction. This intrasocial group came together to help you gain objectivity toward the drama of your fears, your expectations and your self-blame.

Other Driver: I most closely personify the part of you that makes stupid choices out of lack of discernment or unawareness. The reason why I am in this dream is to get you to accept that this is a natural part of yourself and that while you may succeed in reducing it somewhat, it will always be there, so you might as well develop some compassion toward it! This intrasocial group came together to get you to let go of your sense of unfairness or injustice, particularly regarding your relationship with the mother of your daughter.

Dream consciousness: I most closely personify the part of you that loves you enough to put you through pain in order to help you wake up. The reason why I created this dream is to help you let go of your expectations and learn to watch yourself go by. This intrasocial group came together to cultivate your identification with the witness.

Dream Commentary

"If I could change this dream in any way, would I change it? If so, how?"

Ken Wilber:	Knowing what I know now, I would tell the dreamer not to worry about killing me. He can't. I would also tell him to continue to practice listening deeply to himself. That cultivates the witness within him in a moment-to-moment way in his daily life more than meditation does and I know what I'm talking about, because I'm a champion meditator! (But don't get me wrong – I'm not suggesting that he not meditate! On the other hand, you will benefit greatly from practicing at every opportunity!) The weight you want to lose will take care of itself as you learn to listen to your body and to respect what it says it wants and doesn't want.
Girlfriend:	Nothing to add!
Car:	Sounds good to me!
Second Car:	Stop blaming yourself for screwing up!
Other Driver:	Agreed!
Dream consciousness:	Sounds like good advice. I would review the dreamage.
Dream Self:	OK!

(Notice that this Ken Wilber is saying things that the *real* Ken Wilber would not say. Because Wilber is unfamiliar with IDL he would not advocate deep listening over meditation. Even if he was familiar with IDL, he would be unlikely to place a discipline that is anchored in the subtle as higher than a discipline that at best is anchored in the causal and non-dual.)

Dreamage

(A rewrite of the dream based on a consensus of dream group member recommendations. If there is no consensus, there can be no dreamage. A synthesis group dream is usually its own dreamage. Read it over before sleep as an affirmation of a higher pattern of internal integration and healing.)

Ken Wilber and his girlfriend are killed in a head-on car crash. I am very upset. Ken, his girlfriend, their car, the other car, the other driver and myself are all terribly pissed. Some of us indulge in a bit of guilt and self-blame that we allowed this terrible thing to happen. But then we realize that we are all still alive enough to be pissed, so we must not be so dead after all! Now we are figuring out what we need to do to avoid these wrecks in the future. We decide to pray for other drivers and to feel that intent creating mental clarity and purity. We start to get in our cars to continue our lives, but then we decide, after we get to talking, that we are all going in the same basic direction instead of opposite directions. We decide to continue on together in some mutually chosen direction.

Waking Commentary

("If you were the space, the consciousness out of which this dreamer made his daily decisions about how to live his life, how would it be different? How would you handle his three fundamental life issues differently?)

Ken Wilber:	Knowing what I know now, I would tell him not to worry about killing me. He can't. I would also tell him to continue to practice listening deeply to himself. That cultivates the witness within him in a moment-to-moment way in his daily life more than meditation does, and I know what I'm talking about, because I'm a champion meditator! (But don't get me wrong – I'm not suggesting that he not meditate! On the other hand, you will benefit greatly from practicing at every opportunity! The weight will take care of itself as you learn to listen to your body and to respect what it says it wants and doesn't want.
Girlfriend:	Nothing to add!
Car:	Sounds good to me!
Second Car:	Stop blaming yourself for screwing up!
Other Driver:	Agreed!
Dream consciousness:	Sounds like good advice. I would review the dreamage.
Dream Self:	OK!
	(Is there a life issue which you would like to ask these dream group members about?)
Life Issue:	No. This is plenty!

Identification Commentary

Ken Wilber: Become me when you want to cultivate your ability to witness, particularly to gain some objectivity from your addictions in order to become aware of them dispassionately as an aid to their transformation.

Action Plan

(All of these recommendations for waking life applications are not necessarily helpful or of equal importance. You have to decide how you wish to prioritize them and what you want to do with them. But take some action! It is a way of demonstrating that you take

your inner direction seriously. If you have it wrong, future dream groups will cybernetically correct your course.)

General recommendations for fuller application of this dream "reading":

- Regular review of life application of my Action Plan
- Review of this reading
- Regular meditation
- Pre-sleep incubation of my dreamage (if any)
- Pre-sleep incubation of some particular life issue, asking for support of appropriate dream group members.
- Remembering to identify with confident, capable dream group members at specific waking moments, such as when needing more self-acceptance or courage or patience, etc. (Write a list of specific situations where identification with one or another particular dream group member will be particularly helpful, then review how you did at the end of the day.)
- Not to worry about killing myself because I can't!
- Continue to practice listening deeply to myself to cultivate the moment-to-moment witness in my daily life.
- Continue practicing meditation, perhaps with the frame of mind of this Dream Consciousness in mind.
- Listen to my body regarding food preferences.
- Continue to practice being thankful for other drivers.
- I want to take on reviewing the dreamage and practicing being Dream Consciousness at different times during the day, particularly when I am meditating or worried about my weight.

Some of the basic issues addressed by this dream group are

Don't take myself so seriously!

When I screw up, don't waste time beating myself up. It's grandiose to feel so responsible or irresponsible!

Practice thankfulness and appreciation in small ways

"What I am saying to myself is"

(A rewording of comments of dream group members as statements that you are making about yourself.)

(Reword some of the statements made by the dream group members as statements that you are making about yourself to get the full impact of what you are saying to yourself.)

"I am the instrument by which insensitivity and injustice occurs."

"I need to practice non-attachment, thankfulness, appreciation, moment to moment."

"I need to let go of the need to justify my existence."

"I need to drop my unrealistic expectations and my guilt when I don't live up to them."

"I need to let go of my fear of physical death so that I can live more courageously as I grow older."

"I need to learn compassion toward my own self-destruction."

"I need to gain objectivity toward the drama of my fears, my expectations, my self-blame."

"I need to develop some compassion toward the part of myself which makes stupid choices unconsciously out of lack of discernment or unawareness because it is a natural part of myself and it will always be there."

"I need to let go of my sense of my sense of unfairness or injustice, particularly regarding my relationship with Mary Jane."

At this point, what is your understanding of what you think you need to do to be happy in your life?

Sociogram Scoring Key

To determine placement, find the appropriate axis and count one degree of preference for each concentric circle, starting at the center, which is zero.

Positive scores are placed on "+" axes and indicate degree of preference.

Negative scores are placed on "-" axes and indicate degree of rejection.

Vertical (acceptance axis) scores (choosing characters) are taken from the right end of the sociomatrix. This indicates how accepting or rejecting "choosers" are.

Element (chosen characters, actions, and feelings) are taken from the bottom of the sociomatrix. This indicates how preferred or rejected chosen elements are.

Sociogram Commentary

Overall Pattern: This is a strong antithesis pattern with a number of dream group members both rejecting and rejected. It is not a nightmare antithetical pattern because the most nurturing members are still most accepting.

Acceptance Axis: Ken Wilber is the only accepting dream group member. All others are rejecting. Dream Consciousness is most accepting, but it is not a dream group member. The most rejecting dream group member is *Second Car*, presumably because it feels highly victimized.

Form Axis: It is unusual to see an attitude rejected so strongly as is the one personified by "other driver." I really don't like the thoughtless, sleepwalking, negligent, inattentive part of myself! I also don't like the parts of my body that are breaking down and are culpable in my own self-destruction! It's obvious that

Girlfriend and Ken Wilber are both Dream Self surrogates, reinforcing the waking perspectives that puts me in conflict with myself. This teaches me to look beyond the Ken Wilber internal archetype if I want to find integration within myself. It doesn't hold the answer. This is an example of how all gurus have feet of clay and how we all must eventually withdraw our unrealistic projections and expectations about them.

Process Axis: There is no bipolarity here, just widely condemned misbehavior and inattention! There is no internal conflict regarding behavior, because it is all rejected!!!!!

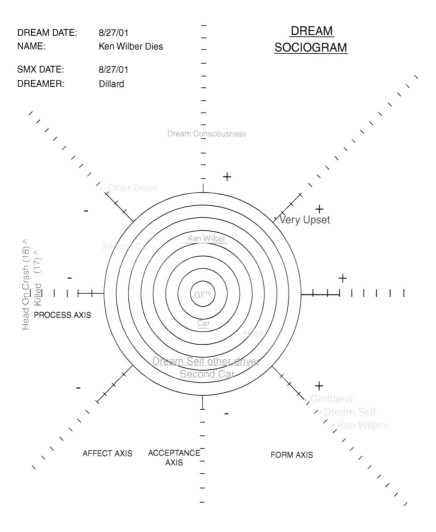

DREAM DATE: 8/27/01
NAME: Ken Wilber Dies

SMX DATE: 8/27/01
DREAMER: Dillard

DREAM
SOCIOGRAM

Dream Consciousness

Other Driver

Very Upset

Head On Crash (18)
Killed   (17)

Ken Wilber

GF

PROCESS AXIS

Car

Dream Self other driver
Second Car

Girlfriend
Dream Self
Ken Wilber

AFFECT AXIS   ACCEPTANCE
AXIS

FORM AXIS

Affect Axis: An uncomfortable behavior is preferred by this dream group because they feel it appropriate to their circumstances, i.e., they identify strongly with victimization.

Dream Group Dynamics Commentary

(In which the various dream group members are provided with an opportunity to express their thoughts on their relationships with their fellow dream group members.)

Ken Wilber: We are not victims of anything but our own unrealistic expectations. If I blame the driver I blame that part of myself which he represents. That's foolish.

Girlfriend: I've got to learn to care big enough to stop caring the way I do!

Car: Hey, cars come and they go. We're here to serve, but when it's time, just let us go!

Second Car: We're imperfect. Don't lose too much sleep over it. Just factor it into your life and make the best of the ride!

Other Driver: I am a part of you and therefore you are destined to screw up. So what? Let go of your unrealistic expectation that you will always be alert, aware, vigilant, discerning, etc., etc. When you fall asleep, just learn from it, give thanks, and go on.

Dream consciousness: I really appreciate the time you took to learn from me.

Dream Self: I give thanks to all these parts of myself for coming together and sacrificing themselves for my greater good. Thank you!

Appendix II
IDL dream interviewing protocol

Joseph Dillard

What are three fundamental life issues that you are dealing with now in your life?

Tell me a dream you remember. It can be an old one, a repetitive dream, a nightmare, or one that you're sure you understand.

Why do you think that you had this dream?

If this dream were playing at a theater, what name would be on the marquee?

These are the characters in the dream, beside yourself . . .

If one character had something especially important to tell you, what would it be?

Now remember how as a child you liked to pretend you were a teacher or a doctor? It's easy and fun for you to imagine that you are this or that character in your dream and answer some questions I ask, saying the first thing that comes to your mind. If you wait too long to answer, that's not the character answering – that's YOU trying to figure out the right thing to say!

_____ are you a character in _____'s dream?

(Character), look out at the world from your perspective and tell us what you see . . .

(Character), would you please tell me about yourself and what you are doing?

(Character), what do you like most about yourself? What are your strengths?

(Character), what do you dislike most about yourself? Do you have weaknesses? What are they?

(Character), what aspect of _____ do you represent or most closely personify?

(Character), what aspect of you does ____ represent or most closely personify?

(Character), if you could be anywhere you wanted to be and take any form you desired, would you change? If so, how?

(Continue, answering as the transformed object, if it chose to change.)

(Character), how would you score yourself 0–10, in each of the following six qualities: confidence, compassion, wisdom, acceptance, inner peace, and witnessing? Why?

Confidence, 0–10. Why?
Compassion, 0–10. Why?
Wisdom, 0–10. Why?
Acceptance, 0–10. Why?
Inner Peace, 0–10. Why?
Witnessing, 0–10. Why?

(Character), if you scored tens in all six of these qualities, would you be different? If so, how?

(Character), how would _____'s life be different if he/she naturally scored like you do in all six of these qualities all the time?

(Character), if you could live _____'s life for him/her, how would you live it differently?

(Character), if you could live _____'s waking life for him/her today, would you handle ____'s three life issues differently? If so, how?

1.
2.
3.

(Character), what life issues would you focus on if you were in charge of _____'s life?

1.
2.
3.

(Character), in what life situations would it be most beneficial for ____ to imagine that he/she is you and act as you would?

(Character), why do you think that you are in _____'s life?

(Character), why do you think _____ had this dream?

(Character), why do you think (some dream event happened) or (some character) was in the dream?

(Character), why should _____ pay any attention to what you have said? Aren't you and your comments just a projection of _____'s own wishes and desires?

Thank you, character! And now a couple questions for _____:

What have you heard yourself say?

If this experience were a wake-up call from your inner compass, what do you think it would be saying to you?

Look back over the interview and list the specific recommendations that were made:

> Every night before you go to sleep read over the recommendations you choose to work on. Score yourself 0–10 on how you did on each. Read the interview over several nights a week to incubate a non-drama alternative reality in your dreams.

Find a partner or a support person, such as another person who you exchange interviews with or an IDL Practitioner. Exchange emails. Send a report each week on how you have done on applying your recommendations. Don't worry about perfection; just focus on making a game out of doing better.

Applying Recommendations for Life Change from Your IDL Interview

1) Make a list of the recommendations in the interview.
2) Choose the ones that you want to work on.
3) Make a weekly chart to track your application daily, before you go to sleep.
4) Operationalize them.

(Write them in a way that change is measurable so that you can test the method. What will be done differently? When?

Are you eating more of this, less of that? Are you thinking different thoughts? Are you feeling different things? Are you talking/acting in different ways to certain people? When? How? What is different?)

5) There will be some items you can check off if you've done them before you go to sleep.
6) Other items need to be rated on a zero to ten scale. How did you do? Rate yourself without criticism. For example:

For example in one interview, Air made a number of suggestions:

I can become Air when I want to not be hungry. It claims that will help, since it doesn't eat.

If I am taking things personally I can become air; it's supposed to help.

Become air to become less mindless or thoughtless.

When having self-doubt, become Air.

Here is an example of how recommendations can be charted daily:

Became Air when: ("v" = less; ^ = more)	M	T	W	Th	F	S	S
hungry	3x	5x	–	3x	4x	6x	–
result (more or less hunger)	v	v	^	v	v	v	^

personalizing	1x	–	–	1x	2x	–	–
result (more or less defensiveness)			v			v	v
mindless	3x	1x	3x	–	–	1x	3x
result (more or less mindful)	^	^	^			^	^
self-doubt	–	–	3x	4x	–	3x	–
result (more or less confidence		^	^		^		

7)   Share your results weekly with someone to create accountability. Have fun!

If you only do a bit of this, no problem. You can come back to this format with successive interviews and over time, you will improve your ability to monitor your application of your recommendations.

Appendix III
IDL life issue interviewing protocol

Joseph Dillard

What are three fundamental life issues that you are dealing with now in your life?

1
2
3

Which issue brings up the strongest feelings for you?

    What feelings does this issue bring up for you?

    If those feelings had a color (or colors), what would it be?

    Imagine that color filling the space in front of you so that it has depth, height, width, and aliveness.

    Now watch that color swirl, congeal, and condense into a shape. Don't make it take a shape, just watch it and say the first thing that you see or that comes to your mind: An animal? Object? Plant? What?

    Now remember how as a child you liked to pretend you were a teacher or a doctor? It's easy and fun for you to imagine that you are the shape that took form from your color and answer some questions I ask, saying the first thing that comes to your mind. If you wait too long to answer, that's not the character answering – that's YOU trying to figure out the right thing to say!

    _____, would you please tell me about yourself and what you are doing?

    (Character), what do you like most about yourself? What are your strengths?

    (Character), what do you dislike most about yourself? Do you have weaknesses? What are they?

    (Character), what aspect of _____ do you represent or most closely personify?

    (Character), what aspect of **you** does your human represent or most closely personify?

    (Character), if you could be anywhere you wanted to be and take any form you desired, would you change? If so, how?

    (Continue, answering as the transformed object, if it chose to change.)

(Character), how would you score yourself 0–10, in each of the following six qualities: confidence, compassion, wisdom, acceptance, inner peace, and witnessing? Why?

Confidence, 0–10. Why?
Empathy, 0–10. Why?
Wisdom, 0–10. Why?
Acceptance, 0–10. Why?
Inner Peace, 0–10. Why?
Witnessing, 0–10. Why?

(Character), if you scored tens in all six of these qualities, would you be different? If so, how?

(Character), how would _____'s life be different if he/she naturally scored like you do in all six of these qualities all the time?

(Character), if you could live _____'s life for him/her, how would you live it differently?

(Character), if you could live _____'s waking life for him/her today, would you handle ____'s three life issues differently? If so, how?

1.
2.
3.

(Character), what life issues would you focus on if you were in charge of _____'s life?

1.
2.
3.

(Character), in what life situations would it be most beneficial for _____ to imagine that he/she is you, become you, and act as you would?

(Character), why do you think that you are in _____'s life?

Thank you, (Character!) Now here are a couple of questions for _____:

What have you heard yourself say?

If this experience were a wake-up call from your inner compass, what do you think it would be saying to you?

Look back over the interview and list the specific recommendations that were made:

Every night before you go to sleep read over the recommendations you choose to work on. Score yourself 0–10 on how you did on each. Read the interview over several nights a week to incubate a non-drama alternative reality in your dreams.

Find a partner or a support person, like another person who you exchange interviews with or an IDL Practitioner. Exchange emails. Send a report each week on how you have done on applying your recommendations. Don't worry about perfection; just focus on making a game out of doing better!

Applying Recommendations for Life Change from Your IDL Interview

1) Make a list of the recommendations in the interview.
2) Choose the ones that you want to work on.
3) Make a weekly chart to track your application daily, before you go to sleep.
4) Operationalize them.

(Write them in a way that change is measurable so that you can test the method. What will be done differently? When?

Are you eating more of this, less of that? Are you thinking different thoughts? Are you feeling different things? Are you talking/acting in different ways to certain people? When? How? What is different?)

5) There will be some items you can check off if you've done them before you go to sleep.
6) Other items need to be rated on a zero to ten scale. How did you do? Rate yourself without criticism. For example:

For example in one interview, Air made a number of suggestions:
I can become Air when I want to not be hungry. It claims that will help, since it doesn't eat.

If I am taking things personally I can become air; it's supposed to help.

Become air to become less mindless or thoughtless.
When having self-doubt, become Air.
Here is an example of how recommendations can be charted daily:

Became Air when: ("v" = less; ^ = more)	M	T	W	Th	F	S	S
hungry	3x	5x	–	3x	4x	6x	-
result (more or less hunger)	v	v	^	v	v	v	^
personalizing	1x	–	–	1x	2x	–	-
result (more or less defensiveness)			v		v	v	
mindless	3x	1x	3x	–	–	1x	3x
result (more or less mindful)	^	^	^			^	^
self-doubt	–	–	3x	4x	–	3x	-
result (more or less confidence		^	^		^		

7) Share your results weekly with someone to create accountability. Have fun!

If you only do a bit of this, no problem. You can come back to this format with successive interviews and over time, you will improve your ability to monitor your application of your recommendations.

Index

For Product Safety Concerns and Information please contact our EU
representative GPSR@taylorandfrancis.com
Taylor & Francis Verlag GmbH, Kaufingerstraße 24, 80331 München, Germany

www.ingramcontent.com/pod-product-compliance
Ingram Content Group UK Ltd.
Pitfield, Milton Keynes, MK11 3LW, UK
UKHW021003180425
457613UK00019B/793